WITHDRAWN-UNL

SUBCELLULAR TAXONOMY

AN ULTRASTRUCTURAL PATHOLOGY PUBLICATION SERIES

Jan Vincents Johannessen and Victor E. Gould, Consulting Editors

McLay and Toner—Subcellular Taxonomy: An Ultrastructural Classification System with Diagnostic Applications

IN PREPARATION

Ingram and Shelburne—Microprobe Analysis in Medicine
Reith and Mayhew—Morphometry and Stereology in Electron Microscopy
Seveus and Roomans—Cryoultramicrotomy

SUBCELLULAR TAXONOMY
an ultrastructural classification system with diagnostic applications

arthur l. c. mclay
University Department of Pathology, Glasgow Royal Infirmary, Scotland

peter g. toner
Department of Pathology, The Queen's University of Belfast, Northern Ireland

○ hemisphere publishing corporation
Washington   New York   London

DISTRIBUTION OUTSIDE THE UNITED STATES
mcgraw-hill international book company
Auckland Bogotá Guatemala Hamburg Johannesburg Lisbon
London Madrid Mexico Montreal New Delhi Panama Paris
San Juan São Paulo Singapore Sydney Tokyo Toronto

SUBCELLULAR TAXONOMY
an ultrastructural classification system
with diagnostic applications

Copyright © 1985 by Hemisphere Publishing Corporation.
All rights reserved. Printed in the United States of America.
Except as permitted under the United States Copyright Act
of 1976, no part of this publication may be reproduced or
distributed in any form or by any means, or stored in a data
base or retrieval system, without the prior written permission
of the publisher.

1 2 3 4 5 6 7 8 9 0   BRBR   8 9 8 7 6 5

This book was set in Univers by Hemisphere Publishing
Corporation. The editors were Christine Flint and Sandra
King; the designer was Sharon Martin DePass; the production
supervisor was Miriam Gonzalez; and the typesetter was
Peggy M. Rote.
Braun-Brumfield, Inc. was printer and binder.

Library of Congress Cataloging in Publication Data

McLay, Arthur L. C., date.
    Subcellular taxonomy.

  (An Ultrastructural pathology publication)
  Bibliography: p.
  Includes index.
    1. Diagnosis, Electron microscopic—Nomenclature.
2. Ultrastructure (Biology)—Nomenclature. I. Toner,
P. G. (Peter G.) II. Title. III. Series. [DNLM:
1. Pathology—Nomenclature. 2. Cells—Ultrastructure—
Nomenclature. 3. Pathology—Nomenclature. QZ 15 M478s]
RB43.5.M34 1983   616.07′582   83-10856
ISBN 0-89116-293-3
ISSN 0730-6482

contents

Preface   vii

ULTRASTRUCTURE, NOMENCLATURE, AND DISEASE

Introduction	3
The Existing SNOMED System	5
Special Problems of Ultrastructural Classification	6
Defects of Existing M-6 and T-YX	7
The Proposed System	9
The Consequences for M-6	10
The Application of the System	13
Specific Problems of Ultrastructural Taxonomy	15
The Role of This System in the Practice of Ultrastructural Pathology	16
Information Retrieval and Computerization	19
Postscript	20
References	21
Selected Readings	21

NUMERICAL LISTING

YX Cellular and Subcellular Structure		25
YX0	The Cell	27
YX1	Nucleus and Associated Structures	27
YX2	Cell Surface and Associated Structures	30
YX3	Cytoplasmic Matrix, Secretory and Metabolic Products	32
YX4	Cytoplasmic Filaments, Tubules, Centrioles, and Associated Structures	33
YX5	Intracytoplasmic Membrane Systems and Associated Structures	35
YX6	Lysosome and Associated Structures. Microbody	37
YX7	Mitochondrion and Associated Structures	38
YX8	Cell to Cell Relationships and Extracellular Structures	39
YX9	Prokaryotic Cell Components	41
YXX	Unclassified	41
YXY	Not Assigned	41

ALPHABETICAL LISTING

A	45	N	70
B	47	O	71
C	49	P	71
D	54	R	74
E	56	S	76
F	58	T	78
G	60	U	79
H	62	V	79
I	62	W	79
J	64	X	79
K	64	Y	79
L	65	Z	80
M	66		

APPENDIX

	Proposed Revised Listing of M-6 Codes	83
600	Karyotype Abnormalities	83
601	Structural Chromosome Alterations	83
603	Centromere Alterations	84
604	Translocations	84
605	Abnormal Chromosome Bandings	84
620	Distinctive Cytologic Morphologies	84
640	Atypia etc.	85
650	Cellular Hormonal Patterns	86

preface

Existing systems of pathologic nomenclature such as the Systematized Nomenclature of Pathology (SNOP) and the Systematized Nomenclature of Medicine (SNOMED) have certain shortcomings when considered for use by the ultrastructural pathologist. In this book an argument is presented that points to the need for a comprehensive system of nomenclature in the field of ultrastructural topography. Detailed proposals for such a system are submitted and its possible uses are outlined. In keeping with standard SNOMED practice the detailed classification has been listed both in numerical and alphabetical form. The system is designed to occupy the T-YX section of SNOMED but could be adapted easily by users of SNOP. Indeed, for certain purposes, this ultrastructural classification can be used independently of any more comprehensive system of nomenclature.

We believe that the system is a practical one, since it has evolved from the needs of a routine ultrastructural pathology service. We anticipate that it may also be of value to experimental pathologists, microbiologists, and anatomists, particularly in the classification, filing, and retrieval of teaching material. We accept that others may see omissions and imperfections that we have overlooked and we hope that interested parties will communicate with us if they have suggestions for its improvement.

We wish to thank Dr. C. G. Gemmel for his advice concerning prokaryotic structures. We are also appreciative of the sustained interest shown in this study by Dr. Roger Côté and Dr. David Rothwell of the SNOMED committee of the College of American Pathologists. Particular thanks are due to Mrs. Marion Thomson for her skill and seemingly limitless patience in typing numerous revisions of this classification. Similarly, thanks are due to Mrs. Isabel Main for typing the later revisions of the central text. Finally, we wish to recognize the support, in the form of equipment grants related to this study, of the Greater Glasgow Health Board Research Support Group and the Scottish Home and Health Department.

Arthur L. C. McLay and Peter G. Toner

ultrastructure, nomenclature, and disease

INTRODUCTION

There has been widespread acceptance by pathologists of the need for some form of systematized nomenclature to provide a basis for the objective and precise classification of different aspects of disease processes. In most departments of pathology, some such system, however primitive, exists for the filing and retrieval of reports issued by the surgical pathology and autopsy services. The value of such systems in case retrieval, retrospective studies, and research collaboration at interdepartmental and international level is self-evident.

For most pathologists, the well-established Systematized Nomenclature of Pathology (SNOP, 1965),[1] with its topographic (T), morphologic (M), etiologic (E), and functional (F) axes, has provided a framework on which filing systems, from the simplest to the most elaborate, have been established. It can be used in its simplest form to provide a two-digit topographic classification for the site of origin of biopsies; it can be used to provide a detailed four-digit morphologic coding of gross and histologic diagnoses; or it can be used to define any combination of topographic, morphologic, etiologic, and functional changes that may be encountered in health care. At one or another of these levels of complexity, SNOP has become an indispensable part of the organization of many departments of pathology. The detailed experience of many users of SNOP confirmed the value of the principle but revealed certain shortcomings in the practical application of the original system, especially in tumor pathology. To deal with these shortcomings, the College of American Pathologists set out to revise SNOP. The outcome of their painstaking work has been the publication of the Systematized Nomenclature of Medicine (SNOMED, 1979).[2] In addition to the four familiar axes of SNOP, three further classifications have been added, a disease axis (D), a procedure axis (P), and an occupation or job axis (J).[3]

These seven axes form a flexible and comprehensive coding structure for all aspects of health care. Some impression of its range and versatility is evident from this, not quite random, selection of codes from the recently published second edition of SNOMED:

T-45000 Artery
T-94000 Carotid body
T-94010 Glomus cell

M-74420 Ichthyosis, acquired
M-50010 Sailor's skin
M-11270 Seaboot foot

E-9115 Motorcycle
E-9152 Kayak
E-9130 Spacecraft

F-01400 Stress, NOS
F-91660 Thinking, lateral
F-Y1170 Defenestration
F-Y1750 Complication of administrative procedure

D-7512 Bagassosis
D-7020 Environment related disease
D-9315 Voodoo

P-0151 Patient referral for consultation
P-0131 Patient transfer to another health care facility, definitive
P-3010 Autopsy

In practice, the universal acceptance of such a system in the wider context of health care may be slow, owing to existing commitments to alternative systems such as ICD (International Classification of Disease, 1977).[4]

The ICD classification, derived from the Bertillon classification of 1893, has been subjected to three revisions since it was adopted by the World Health Organization in 1946. It is a single axis classification that is accepted by most nation members of the Organization for the purpose of publication of health statistics. The single axis limits its versatility and its adaptability as medical science advances. However, as a single list, it is simple to understand and therefore relatively easy to use, even in difficult circumstances in third world countries, where those concerned with operating the system may have limited medical knowledge and certainly limited access to sophisticated facilities for data storage and retrieval. Just as a camel is better adapted to the desert than a Rolls Royce, so, it is argued, ICD may be more appropriate for some purposes in the developing world than a more refined, but much more complex system of classification.

The pathologist, however, has no conflict of loyalties, since no practical alternative to SNOP or SNOMED exists for the purpose of detailed diagnostic coding. In particular ICD is quite inappropriate to this need. There is, therefore, no purpose, at present, in joining the argument concerning the relative merits of SNOMED and ICD over the entire field of health care. Having accepted the need for a system of pathologic nomenclature, we recognize in SNOP and SNOMED the only practical choice. Since SNOMED represents the evolved version of SNOP, we have structured this text around the SNOMED system. Our conclusions and recommendations, however, are equally compatible with SNOP and can quite well stand on their own, independent of any more comprehensive system of nomenclature.

THE EXISTING SNOMED SYSTEM

The pathologist is involved most intimately in the use of the morphologic and topographic fields of SNOMED. The axis of morphology provides a system of five-digit codes under which pathologic processes and diseases can be classified according to their gross and microscopic appearances. It should be noted that the SNOMED definition of morphology is oriented specifically toward abnormal morphology, making the *M* field of SNOMED generally inappropriate for the morphologic description of normality. Strictly speaking, the morphology field might more correctly be termed "pathomorphology."

The axis of topography can be used in a simple two-digit form or in the more complex five-digit form. The purpose of the topographic coding is to identify specific sites, locations, and tissues of the body. It is possible, with a few exceptions, to specify virtually any topographic area, system, organ, tissue, or cell within the body. If desired, the concept of location can then be qualified by the addition of a morphologic concept such as

Normal morphology	*M–00100*
Abnormal appearance	*M–01400*
Increase in size	*M–02510*
Dilatation	*M–32100*

and so on, if circumstances do not require the use of a more specific *M* code such as "inflammation, NOS," *M–40000* to define the pathologic process.

Thus, a typical simple specimen removed during the course of surgery could be represented as follows:

T–66   Appendix
M–41000   Acute inflammation

This particular combination, of course, identifies acute appendicitis. Autopsy coding, although usually covering a wider diagnostic range, is equally straightforward. In a relatively uncomplicated case, wherein death resulted indirectly from rectal carcinoma, the following listing might be appropriate:

T-68	Rectum
M-81403	Adenocarcinoma
M-34000	Obstruction
T-67	Colon
M-32100	Dilatation
T-27900	Terminal bronchiole and lung
M-40000	Bronchopneumonia

More difficult cases would involve the use of additional codes, often including items from the functional and etiologic axes.

SPECIAL PROBLEMS OF ULTRASTRUCTURAL CLASSIFICATION

In ultrastructural pathology, the correlation of specific ultrastructural findings with histology and with the clinical findings in disease is assuming increasing importance.

The role of ultrastructural investigation in the diagnosis of disease, however, is less clearly defined than the role of the light microscope in the parent discipline of histopathology. Over the past hundred years or so, histopathology has evolved through the recognition of increasingly subtle patterns in tissue appearances when viewed in the light microscope. The features thus identified have been extensively catalogued and correlated with clinical outcome, so that a reasonably reliable and comprehensible framework exists for predicting prognosis and choosing appropriate therapy in, perhaps, 80% of cases. In the residual 20% of cases, however, we continue to search for a clearer understanding of the disease process or at least for a pointer toward some related aspect of disease or physiology that we understand better. This is particularly true in tumor diagnosis.

It is in this field, over the past 20 years, that ultrastructural studies have made their most significant contribution. Until recently, such investigations have operated strictly within the framework of existing disease classifications as dictated by the light microscope. More recently, as correlative study has progressed, pathologists engaged in ultrastructural work have come to recognize that the existing framework of tumor nomenclature has significant shortcomings. While in many instances the additional objective criteria provided by the electron microscope reinforce the light microscopic diagnosis, cases increasingly arise in which the findings from the two techniques appear to be at variance with one another. Sometimes the conflict is easily resolved, often by the recognition that certain classic light microscopic patterns are inhomogeneous when viewed at the ultrastructural level. In other cases the conflict is only resolved by the subordination of one set of evidence to the other. Prudence has hitherto tended to favor the established interpretation of light microscopy over conflicting ultrastructural images, the interpretation of which may still be obscure, particularly when the ultrastructural viewpoint is based on a less than systematic analysis. Nevertheless, the ultrastructural dimension cannot be ignored, since it accounts for one third of all recordable morphology. It is now recognized that ultrastructural pathology is a valuable adjunct to conventional histopathology. The challenge is now to bring the interpretation of ultrastructural findings up to the level of sophistication and reliability at which light microscopy presently operates in diagnosis.

When we felt the need for an objective coding system for electron microscopy in the course of our diagnostic work, we turned naturally to SNOMED in an attempt to solve this problem. The compilers of SNOMED, however, in defining their remit, agreed originally to exclude the subcellular dimension from immediate detailed consideration. A separate rank was assigned for subcellular topography (*T-YX*), although this was left largely undeveloped. Subcellular morphology (*M-6*), although treated at slightly greater length, was still seen as a provisional listing. We will now examine these two areas of the existing SNOMED system in greater detail.

DEFECTS OF EXISTING M-6 AND T-YX

The *M-6* rank of SNOMED contains those cellular and subcellular abnormalities that are recognized by the existing system. This rank, however, has several basic weaknesses. At the simplest level, abnormalities of various commonplace subcellular structures such as annulate lamellae, cytoplasmic fibrils, and glycocalyx are not included in the listing. If such a sequence were to be fully effective, it would have to include abnormalities of the entire range of recognized subcellular organelles and structures, without significant omission.

There are, however, more fundamental weaknesses in *M-6* than the lack of codes for abnormalities of specific organelles. From the viewpoint of the ultrastructural pathologist, for example, the nature of the concept of morphology as defined by SNOMED is particularly restrictive. The *M* axis, as has already been mentioned, provides primarily for alterations or abnormalities of structure—pathomorphology. In diagnostic ultrastructural pathology, however, the presence of specific, morphologically normal organelles in tumor cells can be a matter of the greatest diagnostic significance. In a spindle cell tumor, for example, the occurrence of premelanosomes will indicate amelanotic melanoma, while the presence of Weibel-Palade bodies will suggest a diagnosis of angiosarcoma. These are normal anatomic structures rather than subcellular abnormalities, but their identification permits the recognition of differentiation in a tumor that appears undifferentiated by light microscopy. *M-6* fails to recognize this particular problem of ultrastructural pathology.

There is a further weakness in *M-6*. It will be found that many of the entries consist of an abnormality of a specified subcellular component, as in *M-66300,* "Golgi alteration, NOS." Codes such as this are combined codes, incorporating the topographic concept of the specified organelle, along with the morphologic concept of structural abnormality. This is inconsistent with the avowed practice of the SNOMED system, the essence of which is the separation, as far as possible, of topographic and morphologic concepts into their respective axes. There is, for example, no entry elsewhere in SNOMED for "hepatocyte abnormality" or "left kidney abnormality." Instead, there are assorted abnormalities listed under morphology, any of which can be identified as occurring in any topographic location by the use of the appropriate *T* code. For example, the code *M-45000,* "inflammation with fibrosis," can be used in association with *T-96000,* "thyroid gland," to specify Riedel's thyroiditis. The same *M* associated with *T-28010,* "pulmonary alveoli," or *T-31000,* "pericardium," indicates fibrosing alveolitis or adhesive pericarditis, respectively. We believe that the ultrastructural codes should conform to this general rule and that combined codes should be avoided.

Turning to the SNOMED *T* axis, similar problems arise. As mentioned above, the original remit of SNOMED was restricted, for practical reasons, to the histologic and gross classification of disease, leaving subcellular discussion for later development. Thus the rank for cellular and subcellular structure (*T-YX*) permits coding of only 12 subcellular components. It is an incomplete rank with much unused space. A large segment of the existing codes

T-YX 130   Chromosome, NOS
             to
T-YX 167   Chromosomes, group G and Y
             Chromosomes pairs 21–22 and Y

is set aside for the use of the geneticist.

On detailed study of this provisional subcellular classification, we find that few of the structures listed in the combined codes of *M-6* have any corresponding official topographic existence in the *T-YX* sequence. There is, therefore, an "abnormality" of the Golgi apparatus, *M-66300,* but no topographic entity of "Golgi apparatus" in *T-YX*. It became clear to us that the primary problem for the ultrastructural pathologist was the absence, from the SNOMED classification, of a true subcellular topography. For this reason, we set out to produce the system that is listed both numerically and alphabetically in this text.

THE PROPOSED SYSTEM

Bearing in mind the generally adequate range of general morphologic modifiers mentioned above, we concluded that our needs in a diagnostic and research EM unit would be best served by a comprehensive system of ultrastructural topography, supplemented when required by the use of appropriate *M* codes.

Our first efforts in this direction, utilizing an unorthodox *Z* code,[5] were influenced by our familiarity with SNOP and by the fact that the field trial version of SNOMED to which we had access appeared to make no further contribution to the classification of ultrastructural topography. However, following correspondence with Dr. Roger Côté, then Editor-in-Chief of SNOMED, we subsequently recognized that despite the constraint of chromosomal codes for the geneticist, the *T-YX* ranks of the current version of SNOMED (1979) provided the best potential location for our classification, which we then set out to refine and restructure. The resulting classification is based on the main subranks outlined in Table 1 and, as indicated, is listed in full in the Numerical and Alphabetical Listings.

The major subrank headings cover most of the range of subcellular topography likely to be encountered by the pathologist, bacteriologist, and even the general biologist. In the interests of maintaining a coherent, biomedically oriented structure, terms peculiar to plants have been excluded, although with a little ingenuity and the use of the unassigned *YXY* subrank, such a deficiency could readily be remedied by ultrastructural botanists. The chromosomal elements listed in the existing *T-YX* sequence of SNOMED have been incorporated in our subrank *YX1,* nucleus and associated structures, and have, therefore, been subjected to only minor code transposition.

TABLE 1. YX Cellular and Subcellular Structure

YX0	The cell
YX1	Nucleus and associated structures
YX2	Cell surface and associated structures
YX3	Cytoplasmic matrix, secretory and metabolic products
YX4	Cytoplasmic filaments, tubules, centrioles, and associated structures
YX5	Intracytoplasmic membrane systems and associated structures
YX6	Lysosome and associated structures; microbody
YX7	Mitochondrion and associated structures
YX8	Cell to cell relationships and extracellular structures
YX9	Prokaryotic cell components
YXX	Unclassified
YXY	Not assigned

THE CONSEQUENCES FOR M-6

The introduction of a comprehensive topographic listing under *T-YX* has an immediate effect on the existing *M-6* classification of SNOMED. As mentioned above, *M-6* suffers from several basic deficiencies: it is incomplete with regard to its coverage of subcellular components; it does not allow the recording of the occurrence of normal ultrastructural components in, for example, tumors; and it relies extensively on "combined codes," which are against the basic philosophy of the SNOMED system. The first two of these defects are resolved by the introduction of a comprehensive *T-YX* listing. The third defect, the reliance on combined codes, was an inevitable consequence of the absence of a system of ultrastructural topography. It is thus necessary to re-examine the entire *M-6* sequence and to consider what aspects of the listing can now be considered redundant and what should be retained. We have carried out such a review, which is the subject of a submission to the SNOMED committee of the College of American Pathologists. We have eliminated those terms that were considered no longer of value, given an acceptance of our recommendations on *T-YX*. The resulting slim-line *M-6* is listed in full in the Appendix. The following general considerations guided our decisions.

First, we eliminated all terms in *M-6* that were essentially topographic in nature. For example, *M-65020,* "intranuclear dense deposit," was deleted in favor of *T-YX180,* "intranuclear inclusion." *M-65350,* "nucleolar channel system," was deleted in favor of *T-YX175* (identical). *M-67500,* "membrane receptor site, NOS," was deleted in favor of *T-YX842* (identical).

Second, we have eliminated all terms from *M-6* that were clearly "combined codes," incorporating an ultrastructural topographic concept along with a connotation of abnormality. As elsewhere in SNOMED, we recommend the orthodox approach of coding such concepts through the use of paired *T-* and *M-* codes. Thus, *M-63400,* "centromere alteration, NOS," was deleted since it was equivalent to *T-YX128* (centromere) with *M-01000. M-65050,* "nuclear degeneration," was deleted since it was equivalent to *T-YX100* (nucleus) with *M-50000. M-67030,* "plasma membrane rupture," was deleted since it was equivalent to *T-YX200* (cell membrane) with *M-14430.* Third, we eliminated from *M-6* a number of terms that seemed to us to be more correctly handled in the functional (*F*) axis of the SNOMED classification. Thus sections *M-640* and *M-643,* "alterations of genetic material" and "mutations," were transferred en bloc to the *F* listing.

Fourth, we retained in *M-6* those terms that were compatible with a "pure" subcellular pathomorphology, including all of the general cytopathologic terms. Some rearrangement of the retained terms was considered necessary once account was taken of the extensive deletions as detailed above. Thus sections *M-632-633*, "structural chromosomal alterations," and section *M-697*, "cytologic atypias," were retained but restructured and renumbered.

Finally, it became obvious that the accurate recording of subcellular pathology would require a certain number of new terms of a general nature in the *M* sequence. There exists already a group of general *M* terms that can usefully be applied to describe specific abnormalities of subcellular organelles, such as "size decreased" (*M-02520*), "wrinkled" (*M-01450*), and "fusion" (*M-13500*). Other examples can be seen in Table 2. We have added to this list a number of terms that are not at

TABLE 2. *M* Codes for Specific Abnormalities of Subcellular Organelles

00300	Morphology not assigned in SNOMED
00100	Normal morphology
00140	Normal subcellular morphology
00200	Normal size
00360	Normal position
00400	Normal number
00100	Morphologic abnormality, NOS
00110	Lesion, NOS
01110	Minimum lesion
01150	Damage, NOS
01400	Abnormal appearance, NOS
01440	Disruption, NOS
01450	Wrinkled appearance
01460	Compressed structure, NOS
01500	Narrowing, NOS
01520	Obliteration, NOS
01560	Indentation
02000	Shape abnormal, NOS
02500	Size, abnormal, NOS
02510	Size, increased, NOS
02520	Size, decreased, NOS
02540	Asymmetry, NOS
02550	Increase in circumference
02570	Swelling, NOS
02580	Shrinkage, NOS
02590	Contraction, NOS
02600	Thickness, abnormal, NOS
02610	Thickness, increased, NOS
02620	Thickness, decreased, NOS
02960	Opacity, NOS
06000	Normal variation, NOS
09030	Morphologic artefact, NOS
09040	Artefact due to freezing
31100	Shortening, abnormal
31110	Elongation, abnormal
31120	Invagination, NOS
32100	Dilatation, NOS
49400	Adhesion, NOS
50000	Degeneration, NOS
55000	Deposition, NOS

present covered by SNOMED but which we hope can be adopted as new codes under the *M* sequence (Table 3). These will allow greatly increased precision in the classification of ultrastructural pathology but will also, we believe, be of use to histopathologists and other SNOMED users.

As a result of these extensive deletions, the residual *M-6* listing is very short. This should not be taken to imply that subcellular pathology is an undeveloped field, since nothing could be further from the truth. It does, however, reflect our belief that at its present state of evolution, much of subcellular pathology is best expressed in the most basic terms, represented ideally by descriptive *M*-code modifiers of a general nature, applied to specific subcellular topographic entities.

As our understanding of the subcellular milieu increases, truly

TABLE 3. Listing of Proposed New *M* Codes (Not M-6)

Code	Description
01700	Fragmentation
01750	Margination
01800	Rudimentary structure
	Vestigial structure
01900	Mosaicism
02030	Hollow
02010	Folded
02190	Fissured
02130	Fusiform
02230	Tadpole shape
02770	Consistency, granular, NOS
02771	Consistency, granular, coarse
02772	Consistency, granular, fine
050	CHANGES IN QUANTITY
05000	Quantity, abnormal, NOS
05010	Quantity, increased
05020	Quantity, decreased
070–071	CHANGES IN NUMBER
07000	Number, abnormal
07010	Number, increased
	Multiple
07020	Number, decreased
07100	Duplication
07120	Reduplication
080	CHANGES IN DISTRIBUTION
08000	Distribution, abnormal, NOS
08010	Redistribution
08100	Aggregation, NOS
08110	Aggregation, solitary
08120	Aggregation, multiple
08200	Dispersion, NOS
08210	Dispersion, fine
08220	Dispersion, coarse

morphologic information is sure to become more relevant, necessitating the development of a more refined ultrastructural coding in *M-6*. Concise, yet accurate description of the morphologic patterns of relationships between multiple organelles will certainly present problems. Moreover, such refined description is likely to become increasingly remote from the terminology applicable to histopathology, leading to serious problems in correlative study. To draw a historical parallel, similar difficulties might arise in tumor classification during any attempt to harmonize the concepts of Rudolph Virchow with those of Arthur P. Stout.

We would propose an ongoing review of *M-6,* since we would envisage a continuing need for the facilities of both *T-YX* and *M-6* for the ultrastructural pathologist who wishes to achieve the maximum flexibility of classification and recall.

THE APPLICATION OF THE SYSTEM

It is recognized that no simple coordinate system exists for any cell in isolation. This, coupled with the structural lability of the living state, raises theoretical or, rather, philosophical problems as to the true meaning of "subcellular topography." In practice, however, organelles demonstrated in fixed material represent distinctive landmarks within a given cell. In view of the pathomorphologic definition of the *M* axis of SNOMED, to which we have already referred, it was inevitable that the subcellular organelles should fall within the *T* axis.

In a number of instances, such as *T-YX191-194,* "filamentous, granular, and beaded intranuclear bodies," and *T-YX566-567,* "concentric and tubular arrays of GER," our classification verges on what might be termed "topomorphology." On this we are unrepentant, since at this stage the addition of further *M* codes to take account of all such patterns probably represents too great a change in structure. We felt, moreover, that these variations of normal structure were sufficiently distinctive to warrant individual coding. This problem is treated at greater length below.

Although this system is based on SNOMED it is also compatible with SNOP. In SNOP, however, the *YX* rank is already occupied by "peritoneal fluid." SNOP users would therefore need to employ the vacant *YY* rank to accommodate our entire listing. The *YY* rank does not exist in the original SNOP coding, although it is used for temporary individual codes in SNOMED. For those who wish to use this ultrastructural listing independently of any other more general system of nomenclature, the prefix letters could be dropped, leaving a simple three-digit stem as the basis of the entire classification.

The topographic approach that we have adopted involves a coding procedure that is slightly different from the usual *T* and *M* procedure familiar to histopathologists. It is more usual, in pathologic classification, to list a single *T* code, followed perhaps by several detailed *M* codes to describe the identifiable gross and histologic changes of disease. The subcellular classification proposed here is more likely to involve a listing of multiple *T-YX* codes specifying precise subcellular detail, qualified where necessary by a relatively small number of generalized *M* codes representing the type of deviation from normal structure, where this is appropriate. The codes that seem most appropriate in this context are those listed in Tables 2 and 3.

Almost always, these codes will be subordinated to a general *T* and *M* histopathologic coding of the disease process as recognized by existing gross and light microscopic criteria. A typical profile of an unusual but relatively straightforward case might be as follows:

Clear cell gastric neoplasm (bizarre leiomyoma)
- *T-63000* Stomach
- *M-80001* Neoplasm, NOS
- (*M-88911* Epithelioid leiomyoma)
- *T-YX213* Gap junction
- *T-YX803* Cell to cell relationship characterized by alternating areas of cell contact and separation
- *T-YX855* Discontinuous basal lamina
- *T-YX402* Actin-like filaments
- *T-YX418* Dense body, cytoplasmic, with filament insertion

Alternatively, a not entirely dissimilar case presenting significant "histogenetic" problems could be coded in this fashion:

Congenital digital fibroma
- *T-03000* Subcutaneous tissue
- *M-88100* Fibroma, NOS
- *T-YX402* Actin-like filaments
- *T-YX418* Dense body, cytoplasmic, with filament insertion
- *M-01000* Morphologic abnormality, NOS
- (*M-02510* Size increased)
- *T-YX530* Granular endoplasmic reticulum

The myocytic/fibroblastic dualism of this lesion is thus clearly expressed.

This is certainly a difference in tactics, but we believe that it also reflects a real difference in the nature of the exercise of classification between the familiar gross and histologic dimensions on the one hand and the ultrastructural dimension on the other. A useful analogy can be drawn with the image on the screen of a color television set. The picture is constantly changing in its morphology, but at any one moment it can be resolved into an assembly of no more than three basic types of colored dot, the topographic building blocks from which the picture as a whole is made. In the same way, much of the diversity of histopathology can be resolved into patterns built up from a limited number of basic subcellular topographic units.

SPECIFIC PROBLEMS OF ULTRASTRUCTURAL TAXONOMY

In a previous publication[5] that outlined the precursor of the present classification, we recognized that arguments could be made for coding certain subcellular structures in two or more places. In the interests of simplicity it was necessary to make a number of arbitrary allocations. We have adopted the same general approach in the present classification, but the concept of organelle phylogeny has been more rigidly applied. Thus, cilia and flagella, which we previously felt were more appropriately coded under "cell surface and associated components" (YX3) have now been transferred to "cytoplasmic filaments, tubules, centrioles, and associated structures" (YX4) to emphasize their functional relationship to centrioles. Our former viewpoint was based on the assumption that the coding system would be accessed through the numerical listing. Since an alphabetical listing has now been compiled and since we are certain that the most effective access to the system will be through a computer, we have tried to abandon coding in the obvious place in favor of coding in the logical place.

However, as before, certain structural associations were inevitably regarded as of greater importance than strict phylogeny. Thus keratohyalin falls within the YX3 subrank, while the related keratin is found within the YX4 subrank. For similar reasons, the nuclear envelope is in YX1 rather than YX5. The extracellular dense component of the desmosome is such an integral part of the fully developed structure that it logically belongs to YX2 rather than YX8. A similar argument applies to the glycocalyx and intercellular and intracellular canaliculi (YX2), which cannot really be defined without reference to the cell membrane. Among the more arbitrary allocations one might include membrane insertions of filaments in the YX4 rather than the YX2 subrank.

It should be recognized, however, that there are omissions, some of which are quite deliberate. For example, certain aspects of sperm structure were regarded as unique and as having no clearly defined counterpart in other cells. Thus we have not coded for the spermatozoon midpiece, principal piece, endpiece, and the annulus (Jensen's ring). Likewise, we felt that the finer points of the axodendritic or myoneural synapse were beyond the scope of a text such as this; for this reason elements such as the synaptic cleft and puncta adherentia will not be found. Similarly, protozoal microtubular and microfilamentous arrays, such as Km fibers and myonemes, were considered too specialized for inclusion. Having accepted the need for some restraint we have, nevertheless, attempted to include most of the aspects of subcellular structure that are of general occurrence.

THE ROLE OF THIS SYSTEM IN THE PRACTICE OF ULTRASTRUCTURAL PATHOLOGY

In order to give some insight into the use of such a system it is perhaps worthwhile to outline the procedures that we would regard as normal in making an ultrastructural assessment of a surgical biopsy specimen. Any such specimen is accompanied on receipt by a request form (Fig. 1) using Idem paper, which provides multiple copies without carbons. This form permits the recording of basic clinical and technical information concerning the case. The top copy, printed on flimsy paper, accompanies the main record of the case while the second, on light card, is filed in alphabetical sequence. Each case receives a sequence number that is recorded in a daybook together with minimum patient identification data. Each case also has a wallet file that accumulates all diagnostic material related to the case, including micrographs, light microscopic slides, previous reports, and other relevant documentation. When sufficient ultrastructural information is available to the pathologist a report can be generated. This has hitherto taken the form outlined in Fig. 2. It is also executed on Idem paper, this time with three flimsy elements and a light card back. Cases can be coded with ultrastructural *T-YX* codes as well as conventional SNOMED/SNOP codes. The main case wallet is filed in numeric sequence in a filing cabinet, while individual report copies are filed according to one of the related diagnostic codes for the case. Thus, in principle, any case may be retrieved through a variety of routes.

In practice, however, retrieval through the diagnostic codes may prove cumbersome and labor intensive since any individual case is likely to require a greater number of filing locations than is usual in conventional histopathology. For this reason, we have turned to a computerized records system (see next section), which permits greater flexibility in report generation and retrieval.

The capacity to identify cases on the basis of ultrastructural features may have a significant contribution to make in tumor diagnosis. While diagnostic histopathology, at the light microscopic level, is firmly rooted in the scientific basis of medicine, it is, in part, dependent on matching a histologic "wallpaper pattern" with an idealized mental image and is thus somewhat subjective. Although the competent histopathologist can often make a rational analysis to justify a particular diagnosis, few practitioners would deny that they often accept or reject diagnoses with phrases such as "I don't believe it's a . . . , it doesn't feel right."

ULTRASTRUCTURE, NOMENCLATURE, DISEASE 17

Electron Microscopy Request

SPECIMEN NUMBER
SNOP CODE

Nature of Specimen

DATE OF BIRTH   HOSPITAL NO.
FIRST NAME   SURNAME
ADDRESS   SEX/MARITAL STATUS
                OCCUPATION
HOSPITAL   WD/DPT.   CONSULTANT

Collected at   AM/PM.   Date   REPORT REQUESTED BY

Tick box   Surgical Biopsy ☐   Experimental Animal ☐   Autopsy ☐

Clinical History or Experimental Data

LABORATORY DATA

Fixation
Embedding
Grid Box

Histopathology

| Negatives Filed | Transparencies | Demonstration Prints |

Interest	Completion	SNOP	Follow-up
1	2	3	A	B	C	D	E		

FIGURE 1.

Electron Microscopy Report   CASE NUMBER

SNOP CODE

To	Regarding Patient: Hospital Number: Specimen of: Histopathology Reference:

ELECTRON MICROSCOPY UNIT   DEPARTMENT OF PATHOLOGY   GLASGOW ROYAL INFIRMARY

FIGURE 2.

Such subjective views are often most strongly voiced when diagnostic difficulties arise, particularly with tumor groups that appear histologically relatively uniform but in which marked functional diversity is known to occur. A typical example is the spindle cell tumor, which may possess the nature of a squamous cell, a melanocyte, or a connective tissue cell. An analogy might be drawn here from the fine arts. The recognition of patterned diversity within apparent uniformity permits the art connoisseur to identify, for example, individual exponents of the Impressionist school of painting. Bright colors and sophisticated composition enable one to identify Renoir while Monet's hazy patterns and subtleties of light and color are equally distinctive. Yet, while even the interested amateur may find such discrimination relatively easy, only an expert employing every form of assessment, visual and chemical, can be sure of distinguishing the first-class forgery from the old master: the van Meegerin from the Vermeer.

Increasing degrees of objectivity are required for the knowledge that amounts to certainty, and nowhere is this more necessary than where diagnosis is attempted at the limits of conventional histopathology. The identification of subcellular elements together with their functional correlates provides another layer of objectivity, restoring to the histopathologist some power to make a rational analysis in the difficult case. Some organelle patterns are simple and readily recognizable, but the extra information they provide is often so abundant that meaningful patterns are often difficult to discern. It is in this context that computerization of such data may be of value by refining diagnoses through the demonstration of hitherto unsuspected, but recurrent patterns in diagnostic subgroups that may appear uniform by light microscopy.

INFORMATION RETRIEVAL AND COMPUTERIZATION

As indicated in the previous section, the ultrastructural dimension brings with it a dramatic increase in the number of potential markers of differentiation, a matter of considerable importance in tumor pathology. Adequate ultrastructural characterization of a lesion will seldom be possible employing fewer than three or four features. Where more are required and where the pattern formed by the aggregate of such features does not correspond to a distinctive light microscopic diagnosis, significant problems of retrieval are likely to arise. However, where information can be digitized, group matching of selected features is a relatively simple matter for a computer.

In practice we feel that most lesions could be adequately characterized by one general T code, one or two basic M codes, and somewhere between six and twelve T-YX codes. These latter would be supplemented, where necessary, by appropriate modifiers from the general terms in the morphology axis of SNOMED. It is our view that such characterization should be an integral part of a report-generating system based on a dedicated microcomputer with automatic encoding of the appropriate preferred descriptive terms. Broadly speaking, such encoding and retrieval of SNOP/SNOMED related data is already accepted on mainframe/minicomputer systems but has hitherto been regarded as impractical on anything smaller. However, an in house microcomputer system has the advantage of lower capital cost, more economic upgrading in a rapidly developing environment, ease of maintenance and replacement, and, particularly if comprising networked, free-standing units, independence of central processing unit failure.

Our own pilot studies in association with Strathand Ltd.,[*] using a Victor 9000[†] (U.K.—ACT Sirius I), indicate that a comprehensive records system with such a facility is possible with 128 K of random access memory, twin 600 K floppy disc drives, and a 10-megabyte hard

---

[*]Strathand Limited, 2.02 Kelvin Campus, West of Scotland Science Park, Glasgow, G20 0SP, United Kingdom.
[†]Sirius Systems Technology, Inc., Scotts Valley, California.

disc for the long-term storage of compressed data. A complete record would include all patient identification data, surgical pathology accession number, dates of operation and accession, specimen description, and a full report and summary diagnoses with appropriate codes. The size of this record would be approximately 2.5 K and it is stored temporarily on one floppy disc. After delivery to the output terminal (line printer), the final edited report is truncated by the excision of the main report, leaving the surgical pathology number, patient identification data, and the coded data. These truncated data, which occupy 256 bytes of storage capacity, are transferred to a second floppy disc and thence to the hard disc, the second floppy disc serving as a back up. In a data base containing up to 5000 such "short" records, it is estimated that alphabetical and numerical retrieval of case data should be possible within a minute or so, while retrieval on a selection of *T-YX* codes should involve a search time not exceeding 60 minutes.

The quoted speeds of retrieval for alphabetical and numerical data are likely to prove adequate for most ultrastructural diagnostic services in departments of surgical pathology. *T-YX* retrieval, although taking longer, is not likely to present significant problems, since searches of this kind seldom require instant answers and could readily be programmed to operate in batches through lunch hours or overnight. Moreover, these operating limitations are only relevant for the present. Faster search times, easier execution of complex searches, and vastly increased data storage with rapid access are likely in view of the present rapid development of technology in the field of computing. Indeed, random access memory of up to 1.2 megabytes is already practicable in a microcomputer such as we have described.

Such an approach presents new opportunities in the analysis of ultrastructural aspects of disease. It would remain for the ultrastructural pathologist to visualize a plausible subcellular scenario—to develop a hypothesis based on a specific pattern of organelle associations and to test it through retrieval of similar or identical patterns.

POSTSCRIPT

The system just described was devised through the recognition of a diagnostic need within our department. We feel that such a need is likely to exist in similar establishments elsewhere. Should a significant number of centers find it of value, the opportunities for more objective comparisons of interdepartmental ultrastructural data are substantial. However, it seems to us that applications exist outside the framework of a routine diagnostic service. Teaching, both in pathology and anatomy, could benefit significantly from an easily accessible store of ultrastructural data from which specific illustrated features could be drawn. In addition, we feel that when used effectively with *M* modifiers the system has considerable potential for researchers in experimental pharmacology or toxicology.

Taxonomy is usually considered dull and boring and indeed it has its tedious aspects. However, the author/taxonomists of this work, who would be categorized within the framework of SNOMED's occupation codes as *J 05130,* "taxonomist, animal," sometimes found its synthesis light relief from their other occupation, *J 05260,* "medical pathologist." In this latter guise they are often expected by their colleagues to perform tasks more appropriate to *J 17530,* "magician," but equally often in their advocacy of the value of the ultrastructural dimension they feel more like *J 14140,* "evangelist." A voice crying in the wilderness?

REFERENCES

1. Systematized Nomenclature of Pathology (SNOP) Chicago: College of American Pathologists, 1965.
2. Systematized Nomenclature of Medicine (SNOMED). Skokie, Ill.: College of American Pathologists, 1979.
3. Côté RA, Robboy S: Progress in medical information management. Systemized nomenclature of medicine. JAMA 243:756-762, 1980.
4. Manual of the International Statistical Classification of Diseases, Injuries and Causes of Death: Ninth Revision of the International Classification of Diseases. Geneva: World Health Organization, 1977.
5. McLay ALC, Toner PG: Classification of ultrastructural details. Proposals for augmentation of SNOP/SNOMED. Biol Cell 37(1):81-84, 1980.

SELECTED READINGS

Carr KE, Toner PG: Cell Structure, 3d ed. London: Churchill-Livingstone, 1982.
Fawcett DW: The Cell, 2d ed. Philadelphia: Saunders, 1981.
Ghadially FN: Diagnostic Electron Microscopy of Tumours. London: Butterworths, 1980.
Ghadially FN: Ultrastructural Pathology of the Cell and Matrix, 2d ed. London: Butterworths, 1982.
Henderson DW, Papadimitriou JM: Ultrastructural Appearances of Tumours. London: Churchill-Livingstone, 1982.
Johannessen JV (ed): Electron Microscopy in Human Medicine, Vols. 1-10. New York: McGraw-Hill, 1978-1982.
Kristic RV: Ultrastructure of the Mammalian Cell. New York: Springer-Verlag, 1982.
McLay ALC, Toner PG: Diagnostic electron microscopy. In: Recent Advances in Histopathology, 11th ed, edited by PP Anthony, RNM MacSween. London: Churchill-Livingstone, 1981.
Trump BF, Jones RT (eds): Diagnostic Electron Microscopy, Vols. 1-3. New York: Wiley, 1978-1980.

numerical listing

yx cellular and subcellular structure

YX0   The cell

YX1   Nucleus and associated structures

YX2   Cell surface and associated structures

YX3   Cytoplasmic matrix, secretory and metabolic products

YX4   Cytoplasmic filaments, tubules, centrioles, and associated structures

YX5   Intracytoplasmic membrane systems and associated structures

YX6   Lysosome and associated structures. Microbody

YX7   Mitochondrion and associated structures

YX8   Cell to cell relationships and extracellular structures

YX9   Prokaryotic cell components

YXX   Unclassified

YXY   Not assigned

YX0   The cell

YX000	Cell, NOS
YX001	Subcellular structure, NOS
YX002	Subcellular structure, isolated by fractionation technique
YX010	Central region of cell
YX011	Centrosome
YX112	Perinuclear region of cell
YX013	Peripheral region of cell
YX014	Apical region of polarized cell
YX015	Lateral region of polarized cell
YX016	Supranuclear region of polarized cell
YX017	Infranuclear region of polarized cell
YX018	Basal region of polarized cell
YX020	Dividing cell, NOS
YX030	Mitotic cell, NOS
YX031	Mitotic cell in prophase
YX032	Mitotic cell in metaphase
YX033	Mitotic cell in anaphase
YX034	Mitotic cell intelophase
YX035	Anaphase constriction
YX036	Telophase midbody
YX040	Meiotic cell, NOS

YX1   Nucleus and associated structures

YX100	Nucleus, NOS
YX101	Interphase nucleus
YX102	Mitotic nucleus, NOS
YX103	Prophase nucleus
YX104	Metaphase nucleus
YX105	Metaphase plate
YX106	Anaphase nucleus
YX107	Telophase nucleus
YX110	Nuclear envelope, NOS
	Karyotheca
YX111	Nuclear envelope, evagination
	Nuclear bleb
YX112	Nuclear envelope, outer membrane
YX113	Nuclear envelope, outer membrane evagination
YX114	Nuclear envelope, inner membrane

YX115	Nuclear envelope, invagination
	Cytoplasmic pseudo-inclusion
YX116	Perinuclear cisterna
	Perinuclear space
YX117	Nuclear pore apparatus
YX118	Diaphragm, nuclear pore
YX119	Nuclear fibrous lamina
YX120	Chromatin, NOS
	Karyoplasm
	Nuclear sap
YX121	Perinucleolar chromatin
YX122	Euchromatin
	Chromatin extended
YX123	Heterochromatin
	Chromatin condensed
YX124	Perichromatin granule
YX125	Interchromatin granule
YX126	Sex chromatin
	Barr body
YX127	Chromatid, NOS
YX128	Centromere
YX129	Kinetochore
YX130	Chromosome, NOS
YX131	Chromosome pair 1
YX132	Chromosome pair 2
YX133	Chromosome pair 3
YX134	Chromosome pair 4
YX135	Chromosome pair 5
YX136	Chromosome pair 6
YX137	Chromosome pair 7
YX138	Chromosome pair 8
YX139	Chromosome pair 9
YX140	Chromosome pair 10
YX141	Chromosome pair 11
YX142	Chromosome pair 12
YX143	Chromosome pair 13
YX144	Chromosome pair 14
YX145	Chromosome pair 15
YX146	Chromosome pair 16
YX147	Chromosome pair 17
YX148	Chromosome pair 18
YX149	Chromosome pair 19
YX150	Chromosome pair 20

YX151	Chromosome pair 21
YX152	Chromosome pair 22
YX153	Chromosome pair 23
YX159	Sex chromosome, NOS
YX15X	Sex chromosome X
YX15Y	Sex chromosome Y
YX160	Chromosome group, NOS
YX161	Chromosomes, group A
	Chromosome pairs 1-3
YX162	Chromosomes, group B
	Chromosome pairs 4-5
YX163	Chromosomes, group C & X
	Chromosome pairs 6-12 & X
YX164	Chromosomes, group D
	Chromosome pairs 13-15
YX165	Chromosomes, group E
	Chromosome pairs 16-18
YX166	Chromosomes, group F
	Chromosome pairs 19-20
YX167	Chromosomes, group G & Y
	Chromosome pairs 21-22 & Y
YX170	Nucleolus, NOS
YX171	Nucleolonema of nucleolus
	Pars granulosa of nucleolus
YX172	Pars amorpha of nucleolus
	Pars fibrosa of nucleolus
YX173	Nucleolinus
	Fibrillar center of nucleolus
YX174	Nucleolar cap
YX175	Nucleolar channel system
YX180	Intranuclear inclusion, NOS
YX181	Intranuclear cell product (F-...)
YX182	Intranuclear crystal
	Crystalline inclusion, intranuclear
YX183	Intranuclear filaments
	Filamentous inclusion, intranuclear
YX184	Intranuclear membrane lamellae
	Lamellar inclusion, intranuclear
YX185	Intranuclear tubule
	Tubular inclusion, intranuclear
YX186	Intranuclear glycogen
YX187	Intranuclear lipid
YX188	Intranuclear secretory granule

YX189	Intranuclear mitochondrion
YX190	Intranuclear body, NOS
	Nuclear body
YX191	Intranuclear body, filamentous
	Simple nuclear body
YX192	Intranuclear body, granular with filamentous capsule
YX193	Intranuclear body, beaded intranuclear filaments
YX194	Intranuclear body, concentrically laminated
YX195	Intranuclear body, rod shaped

YX2   Cell surface and associated structures

YX200	Cell membrane, NOS
	Plasmalemma
	Plasma membrane
YX201	Cell membrane, apical aspect of polarized cell
YX202	Cell membrane, lateral aspect of polarized cell
YX203	Cell membrane, basal aspect of polarized cell
YX204	Fractured membrane E face
YX205	Fractured membrane P face
YX206	Fractured membrane particle
YX207	Fractured membrane particle array
YX208	Connexon
YX209	Dense zone, internal aspect of cell membrane, not desmosome
YX210	Cell adhesion specialization, NOS
YX211	Junctional complex, NOS
YX212	Tight junction
	Close junction
	Zonula occludens
YX213	Gap junction
	Nexus
YX214	Intermediate junction
	Zonula adherens
YX215	Desmosome
	Macula adherens
YX216	Autodesmosome
YX217	Intracytoplasmic desmosome
YX218	Hemidesmosome
YX219	Extracellular dense component of desmosome or hemidesmosome
YX220	Adhesion specialization in functionally specialized tissue, NOS
YX221	Desmosome of mature keratinocyte
	Cementsome (T-01152)

YX222	Intercalated disc of myocardium (T-33101)
YX223	Synaptic membrane specialization, NOS
YX224	Synaptic membrane specialization, presynaptic
YX225	Synaptic membrane specialization, postsynaptic
YX226	Septate junction
	Septate desmosome
YX230	Cell process, NOS
YX231	Microvillus
YX232	Striated border
YX233	Stereocilium
YX234	Filipodium
YX235	Lamellipodium
	Ruffle
YX236	Uropod
YX237	Vermipodium
YX238	Axopod
YX240	Distinctive surface process of specialized cell, NOS
YX241	Marginal fold of endothelial cell (T-05130)
YX242	Foot process of glomerular podocyte, NOS (T-71200)
YX243	Primary foot process (T-71200)
YX244	Secondary foot process (T-71200)
	Pedicel
YX245	Slit pore of glomerular podocyte (T-71200)
YX246	Sensory hair (T-XY840, T-XY890)
YX250	Fenestration, endothelial, NOS (T-05130)
YX251	Fenestration, endothelial, with diaphragm (T-05130)
YX252	Fenestration, endothelial, without diaphragm (T-05130)
YX253	Diaphragm of fenestration (T-05130)
YX254	Sieve plate, endothelial (T-05130)
YX260	Membrane invagination, fixed or stable, NOS
YX261	Basal infolding of cell membrane
YX262	Intracellular canaliculus
YX263	Intercellular canaliculus
YX264	T tubule of striated muscle
YX265	Intracytoplasmic lumen
YX270	Membrane invagination, labile, NOS
YX271	Membrane invagination, labile, endocytic
YX272	Membrane invagination, labile, exocytic
YX273	Micropinocytotic vesicle, NOS
	Caveola
YX274	Simple caveola
YX275	Coated vesicle
	Acanthosome
	Fuzzy vesicle

YX276	Rhopheocytotic vesicle
YX277	Micropinocytosis vermiformis channel
YX278	Content of endocytic membrane invagination (T–YX . . . or F– . . .)
YX279	Content of exocytic membrane invagination (F– . . .)

YX280	Glycocalyx, NOS
	    Cell coat
	    Fuzzy coat

YX281	Distinctive form of glycocalyx, NOS
YX282	Antennulae microvillares
YX283	Cuticle of cell
YX284	Membrane receptor (F– . . .)
YX290	Distinctive form of cell envelope, NOS
YX291	Cell wall, eukaryotic
YX292	Pellicle, as in protozoal parasite

YX3 Cytoplasmic matrix, secretory and metabolic products

YX300	Cytoplasmic matrix, NOS
	    Cytoplasm
	    Hyaloplasm

YX310	Cytoplasmic inclusion, NOS
YX311	Cytoplasmic inclusion, crystalline
YX312	Cytoplasmic inclusion, paracrystalline
YX313	Cytoplasmic inclusion, granular
YX314	Cytoplasmic inclusion, filamentous
YX320	Cytoplasmic vacuole, NOS, not related to GERL
YX330	Secretory granule, NOS
YX331	Secretory granule, exocrine, NOS
YX332	Secretory granule, exocrine, known content (F– . . .)
YX333	Secretory granule, exocrine, undergoing exocytosis
YX334	Secretory granule, exocrine, known content (F– . . .) undergoing exocytosis
YX335	Mucus granule
YX336	Zymogen granule
YX340	Secretory granule, endocrine, NOS
YX341	Secretory granule, endocrine, known content (F– . . .)
YX342	Secretory granule, endocrine, undergoing exocytosis
YX343	Secretory granule, endocrine, known content (F– . . .) undergoing exocytosis
YX344	Neurosecretory granule
YX345	Synaptic vesicle, NOS

YX346	Dense-cored synaptic vesicle
YX350	Distinctive cytoplasmic granule of specialized cell (T- . . .)
YX351	Melanogenic granule, NOS
YX352	Premelanosome
YX353	Melanosome, incompletely melanized
YX354	Melanosome, completely melanized
	Melanin granule
YX355	Complex melanin-containing granule
YX356	Langerhans granule
	Birbeck granule
YX357	Lamellated granule, as in surfactant-secreting cell
	Cytosome
YX360	Endothelial cell granule
	Weibel-Palade granule
YX361	Keratohyaline granule
YX362	Membrane-coating granule, NOS
	Odland body
YX363	Membrane-coating granule, laminated
YX364	Membrane-coating granule, amorphous
YX370	Cytoplasmic metabolite, structurally distinctive, NOS
YX371	Glycogen, NOS
YX372	α Glycogen
YX373	β Glycogen
YX374	Ferritin
YX380	Lipid droplet, NOS
YX381	Lipid droplet, homogeneous
YX382	Lipid droplet, lamellated
YX383	Lipid droplet, complex
YX384	Lipid, crystalline
	Cholesterol crystal

YX4   Cytoplasmic filaments, tubules, centrioles, and associated structures

YX400	Cytoplasmic filaments, NOS
YX401	Filaments of contractile apparatus, NOS
	Myofilaments
YX402	7nm filaments
	Actin-like filaments
YX403	12nm filaments
	Myosin-like filaments
YX404	Combined actin-like and myosin-like filaments
YX405	Distinctive arrangement of cytoplasmic filaments, NOS

YX410	Sarcomere pattern, NOS
YX411	*A* band
YX412	*I* band
YX413	*H* zone
YX414	*M* line
YX415	*Z* line
YX416	*Z* line material
YX417	Filament insertion into cytoplasmic dense body
YX418	Filament insertion into cytoplasmic dense body
YX419	Filament insertion into dense zone on internal aspect of cell membrane, not desmosome
YX420	Structural filaments, NOS

YX421	9nm filaments
	    Intermediate filaments
	    Tonofilaments

YX422	Diffuse tonofilaments
YX423	Dense intermediate filament bundles Tonofibrils
YX424	Tonofilaments related to desmosome or hemidesmosome Filament insertion into desmosome or hemidesmosome
YX425	Attachment plaque of desmosome or hemidesmosome
YX426	Intermediate filaments of known composition (F- . . .)
YX427	Mature keratin
YX430	Cytoplasmic microtubule, NOS
YX431	Distinctive arrangement of microtubules, NOS
YX432	Marginal band of microtubules
YX433	Microtubules associated with cytoplasmic filaments Cytoskeleton
YX434	Microtubules associated with cell organelle (T-YX . . .)
YX435	Adhesion disc of parasite
YX440	Mitotic spindle, NOS
YX441	Continuous microtubules of spindle
YX442	Interzonal microtubules of spindle
YX443	Pole of spindle
YX450	Centriole, NOS
YX451	Centriole, microtubular subunit Triplet
YX452	Centriole, central vesicle
YX453	Procentriole
YX454	Satellite, centriolar
YX455	Basal body of cilium or flagellum, not bacterial Kinetosome
YX456	Rootlet of cilium or flagellum, not bacterial

YX460	Cilium, NOS
	Kinocilium
YX461	Rudimentary cilium
YX462	Flagellum, not bacterial, NOS
YX463	Shaft of cilium or flagellum, not bacterial
YX464	Membrane of cilium or flagellum, not bacterial
YX465	Axial filament complex, NOS, of cilium or flagellum, not bacterial
	Axoneme
	Axonemal complex
YX466	Peripheral microtubular doublet of cilium or flagellum, not bacterial
YX467	Subunit *a* of peripheral doublet of cilium or flagellum, not bacterial
YX468	Subunit *b* of peripheral doublet of cilium or flagellum, not bacterial
YX469	Dynein arm of peripheral doublet of cilium or flagellum, not bacterial
YX470	Central pair of microtubules, cilium or flagellum, not bacterial
YX471	Solitary microtubule component of centriole or axonemal complex
	Singlet
YX480	Specialized cilium or flagellum, NOS
YX481	Sensory cilium, olfactory (T-X8020)
YX482	Retinal photoreceptor, outer segment (T-XX610)
YX490	Specialized subunit or derivative of cilium or flagellum, not bacterial, NOS
YX491	Fibrous sheath of sperm tail (T-78180)

YX5   Intracytoplasmic membrane systems and associated structures

YX500	GERL, NOS
YX510	Golgi complex, NOS
	Golgi apparatus
	Golgi system
YX511	Golgi membrane
YX512	Golgi saccule
YX513	Golgi vacuole
	Condensing vacuole
YX514	Golgi vesicle, NOS

YX515	Transport vesicle of Golgi complex
	Transitional vesicle
YX516	Inclusion within Golgi complex
YX520	Endoplasmic reticulum, NOS
	ER
YX521	Endoplasmic reticulum, NOS, membrane
YX522	Endoplasmic reticulum, NOS, cisternal lumen
YX523	Confronting cisternae of ER
YX524	Endoplasmic reticulum, NOS, connection with other organelle (T-YX . . .)
YX525	Intracisternal material, NOS
YX526	Intracisternal material, amorphous
YX527	Intracisternal material, periodic
YX528	Intracisternal granule of ER, NOS
YX529	Intracisternal material of known identity (F- . . .)
YX530	Granular endoplasmic reticulum (GER), NOS
YX531	Granular endoplasmic reticulum membrane
YX532	Granular endoplasmic reticulum, cisternal lumen
YX533	Granular endoplasmic reticulum, connection with other organelle (T-YX . . .)
YX540	Ribosome, NOS
YX541	Ribosome, free in cytoplasm
YX542	Ribosome, attached to GER membrane
YX543	Ribosome, attached to outer nuclear membrane
YX544	Polyribosome, NOS
YX545	Polyribosome, free in cytoplasm
YX546	Polyribosome, attached to GER membrane
YX547	Polyribosome, attached to outer nuclear membrane
YX550	Agranular endoplasmic reticulum, NOS
	AER
	SER
	Smooth endoplasmic reticulum
YX551	Agranular endoplasmic reticulum membrane
YX552	Agranular endoplasmic reticulum, cisternal lumen
YX553	Agranular endoplasmic reticulum, connection with other organelle (T-YX . . .)
YX560	Distinctive arrangement or relationship of endoplasmic reticulum, NOS
YX561	ER related to cell surface
YX562	ER related to mitochondrion
YX563	ER related to other cell component (T-YX . . .)
YX564	GER aggregate, NOS
	Ergastoplasm
	Nissl granule
	Nissl substance

YX565	GER concentric array
YX566	GER tubular array
YX567	AER aggregate, NOS
YX568	AER of striated muscle
	Sarcoplasmic reticulum
YX569	Triad of striated muscle
YX570	Annulate lamella, NOS
YX571	Annulate lamella, membrane
YX572	Annulate lamella, cisternal lumen
YX573	Annulate lamella, fenestration
YX574	Annulate lamella, diaphragm of fenestration
YX580	Distinctive intracytoplasmic membrane system, not Golgi complex or ER
YX581	Photoreceptor membrane lamellae
YX582	Fusiform vesicle, as in transitional epithelium
YX590	Synaptic specialization, cytoplasmic, NOS
YX591	Dendritic spine apparatus

YX6   Lysosome and associated structures. Microbody

YX600	Lysosome, NOS
YX601	Membrane of lysosome
YX602	Matrix of lysosome
YX610	Primary lysosome, NOS
YX620	Secondary lysosome, NOS
YX621	Heterolysosome
	Phagolysosome
	Phagosome
YX622	Secondary lysosome with distinctive content (T--YX . . . or F- . . .)
YX623	Secondary lysosome with laminated content
	Myelin figure, lysosome-derived
YX624	Secondary lysosome with ferritin content
	Siderosome
YX625	Secondary lysosome undergoing exocytosis
YX626	Residual body
	Lipofuscin granule
	Telolysosome
YX627	Adhesion specialization between lysosomes
YX630	Autolysosome, NOS
	Autophagocytic vacuole
	Cytolysosome
	Cytosegresome
	Focal cytoplasmic degeneration

YX631	Autolysosome containing recognizable cytoplasmic organelle (T-YX . . .)
YX632	Autolysosome containing secretion granule (F- . . .)
	Crinophagocytic vacuole
YX640	Multivesicular body, NOS
	Vesicle-containing body
YX641	Multivesicular body, surrounding membrane
YX642	Multivesicular body, internal vesicles
YX643	Multivesicular body, inclusion
YX650	Lysosome of male germ cell (T-78180)
	Acrosome
YX651	Acrosomal granule (T-78170)
YX652	Proacrosomal granule (T-78170)
YX653	Acrosomal vesicle (T-78170)
YX660	Microbody, NOS
	Peroxisome
YX661	Microbody membrane
YX662	Microbody matrix
YX663	Microbody nucleoid, NOS
YX664	Microbody nucleoid, amorphous
YX665	Microbody nucleoid, periodic
YX666	Adhesion specialization between microbodies

YX7   Mitochondrion and associated structures

YX700	Mitochondrion, NOS
YX701	Mitochondrial membrane, outer
YX702	Mitochondrial membrane, inner
YX703	Mitochondrial membrane particle
	Electron transport particle
YX704	Mitochondrial space, outer
YX705	Mitochondrial space, inner
	Mitochondrial matrix
YX706	Mitochondrial cristae
YX707	Adhesion specialization between mitochondria
YX708	Mitochondrial "bridge"
YX710	Distinctive shape of mitochondrial cristae, NOS
YX711	Fenestrated cristae of mitochondrion
YX712	Tubular cristae of mitochondrion
YX713	Branching cristae of mitochondrion
YX714	Saccular cristae of mitochondrion

YX715	Prism-shaped cristae of mitochondrion
YX720	Distinctive pattern of mitochondrial cristae, NOS
YX721	Close packing of cristae of mitochondrion
YX722	Transverse orientation of cristae of mitochondrion
YX723	Longitudinal orientation of cristae of mitochondrion
YX724	Concentric orientation of cristae of mitochondrion
YX725	Zig-zag configuration of cristae of mitochondrion
YX730	Mitochondrial inclusion, NOS
YX731	Mitochondrial matrix inclusion, NOS
YX732	Intramitochondrial granule Matrix granule
YX733	Intramitochondrial crystal
YX734	Intramitochondrial DNA
YX735	Intramitochondrial ribosome
YX740	Intramitochondrial cell metabolite (F-...)
YX741	Intramitochondrial ferritin
YX742	Intramitochondrial lipid
YX750	Mitochondrial aggregation within cytoplasm, NOS
YX751	Mitochondrial association with other cell component (T-YX...)
YX752	Chondriosphere
YX760	Mitochondrion in division
YX770	Kinetoplast, NOS
YX780	Plastid, NOS

YX8   Cell to cell relationships and extracellular structures

YX800	Cell to cell relationship, distinctive, NOS
YX801	Cell to cell relationship, characterized by cell separation, contact minimal or absent
YX802	Cell to cell relationship, characterized by focal cell contact
YX803	Cell to cell relationship, characterized by alternating areas of cell contact and separation
YX804	Cell to cell relationship, characterized by cell contact, separation minimal or absent
YX805	Cell to cell relationship, characterized by interdigitation
YX806	Cell to cell relationship, characterized by absence of adhesion specializations
YX807	Cell to cell relationship, characterized by scantiness of adhesion specializations
YX808	Cell to cell relationship, characterized by presence of adhesion specializations

YX809	Cell to cell relationship, characterized by abundance of adhesion specializations
YX810	Extracellular space, NOS
YX811	Intercellular space, NOS
YX812	Complex or labrynthine intercellular space
YX820	Extracellular material, NOS
YX821	Extracellular metabolic product (F-...)
YX822	Extracellular secretion material following exocytosis, luminal (exocrine secretion)
YX823	Extracellular secretion material following exocytosis, interstitial (endocrine secretion)
YX824	Extracellular lipid droplet
	Chylomicron
YX830	Connective tissue matrix, NOS
YX831	Diffusely mineralized extracellular matrix
YX832	Focally mineralized extracellular matrix
YX833	Non-mineralized extracellular matrix
YX834	Extracellular crystal
YX835	Amorphous or granular extracellular material
YX836	Fibrin
YX840	Connective tissue fiber, NOS
YX841	Collagen fibrils, 64nm spacing
YX842	Long spacing collagen fibrils
YX843	Collagen protofibrils
YX844	Elastic fiber, NOS
YX845	Elastic fiber, amorphous component
YX846	Elastic fiber, microfilamentous component
YX847	Connective tissue microfibrils
YX850	Basal lamina, NOS
	Basement membrane
	External lamina
YX851	Basal lamina of epithelial cell or tissue
YX852	Basal or external lamina of non-epithelial cell or tissue
YX853	Basal or external lamina of specialized cell or tissue (T-...)
YX854	Mesangial matrix (T-71290)
YX855	Discontinuous or incomplete basal or external lamina
YX856	Basal lamina, lamina densa component
YX857	Basal lamina, lamina rara interna component
YX858	Basal lamina, lamina rara externa component
YX859	Basal lamina, anchoring filaments
YX860	Basal lamina, inclusion, NOS
YX861	Basal lamina, inclusion consisting of cell process
YX862	Basal lamina, inclusion consisting of dense deposit
YX863	Basal lamina, inclusion in central location
YX864	Basal lamina, inclusion in subendothelial location

YX865	Basal lamina, inclusion in subepithelial location
YX866	Mesengial matrix inclusion (T-71290; T-YX854)

YX9 Prokaryotic cell components

YX900	Cell capsule, prokaryotic, NOS
YX901	Macrocapsule
YX902	Microcapsule
YX910	Cell wall, prokaryotic, NOS
YX911	Cell wall, prokaryotic, Gram +ve organism
YX912	Cell wall, prokaryotic, Gram −ve organism
YX913	Cell wall, prokaryotic, septum
YX914	Surface convolutions of cell wall
YX920	Flagellum, bacterial, NOS
YX921	Flagellum, bacterial, shaft
YX922	Flagellum, bacterial, basal structure
YX930	Pilum, NOS
	Fimbria
YX931	Common pilum
YX932	Sex pilum
YX940	Cell membrane, prokaryotic, NOS
YX941	Protoplast membrane
YX942	Mesosome
YX950	Cell contents, prokaryotic, NOS
YX951	Cytoplasm, prokaryotic
YX952	Nuclear material, prokaryotic
YX953	Ribosome, prokaryotic
YX954	Granular inclusion, prokaryotic
YX960	Spore structure, NOS
YX961	Fore spore membrane
YX962	Spore outer coat
YX963	Spore cortex
YX964	Spore inner coat
YX965	Spore cytoplasmic membrane
YX966	Spore cytoplasm
YX967	Spore crystal

YXX Unclassified

YXX00	Unclassified ultrastructural features, NOS

YXY Not assigned

alphabetical listing

a

YX372	α Glycogen
YX411	*A* band, sarcomere
YX275	Acanthosome
YX651	Acrosomal granule (T-78170)
YX653	Acrosomal vesicle (T-78170)
YX650	Acrosome (T-78180)
YX402	Actin-like filaments, 7nm
YX435	Adhesion disc of parasite
YX220	Adhesion specialization in functionally specialized tissue, NOS
YX210	Adhesion specialization of cell, NOS
YX806	Adhesion specializations between cells absent
YX809	Adhesion specializations between cells abundant
YX808	Adhesion specializations between cells present
YX807	Adhesion specializations between cells scanty
YX666	Adhesion specialization between microbodies or peroxisomes
YX627	Adhesion specialization, lysosomal
YX607	Adhesion specialization, mitochondrial
YX550	AER (SER), NOS
YX567	AER (SER), aggregate, NOS
YX553	AER (SER), connection with other organelle (T-YX . . .)
YX568	AER (SER), striated muscle
YX567	Aggregate of AER (SER), NOS
YX564	Aggregate of GER (RER), NOS
YX750	Aggregation of mitochondria within cytoplasm, NOS
YX567	Agranular endoplasmic reticulum aggregate, NOS
YX552	Agranular endoplasmic reticulum cisternal lumen
YX553	Agranular endoplasmic reticulum, connection with other organelle (T-YX . . .)

YX551	Agranular endoplasmic reticulum membrane
YX550	Agranular endoplasmic reticulum, NOS
YX568	Agranular endoplasmic reticulum, striated muscle
YX845	Amorphous component of elastic fiber
YX835	Amorphous extracellular material
YX526	Amorphous material within ER cisterna
YX364	Amorphous membrane-coating granule
YX664	Amorphous nucleoid of microbody or peroxisome
YX035	Anaphase constriction
YX033	Anaphase, mitotic cell
YX106	Anaphase nucleus
YX859	Anchoring filaments, basal lamina
YX572	Annulate lamella, cisternal lumen
YX573	Annulate lamella, fenestration
YX574	Annulate lamella, diaphragm of fenestration
YX571	Annulate lamella membrane
YX570	Annulate lamella, NOS
YX282	Antennulae microvillares
YX201	Apical cell membrane, polarized cell
YX014	Apical region, polarized cell
YX591	Apparatus, dendritic spine
YX510	Apparatus, Golgi, NOS
YX117	Apparatus, nuclear pore
YX565	Array, concentric, GER (RER)
YX207	Array of particles in fractured membrane
YX566	Array, tubular, GER (RER)
YX201	Aspect, apical, polarized cell, cell membrane
YX203	Aspect, basal, polarized cell, cell membrane
YX202	Aspect, lateral, polarized cell, cell membrane
YX425	Attachment plaque of desmosome or hemidesmosome
YX216	Autodesmosome
YX631	Autolysosome containing recognizable cytoplasmic organelle (T-YX . . .)
YX632	Autolysosome containing secretion granule (F- . . .)
YX630	Autolysosome, NOS
YX630	Autophagocytic vacuole, NOS
YX465	Axial filament complex, NOS, of cilium or flagellum, not bacterial
YX465	Axonemal complex
YX471	Axonemal complex, solitary microtubule component
YX465	Axoneme
YX238	Axopod

b

YX373	β Glycogen
YX900	Bacterial cell, capsule, NOS
YX931	Bacterial cell, common pilum
YX950	Bacterial cell, contents, NOS
YX951	Bacterial cell, cytoplasm
YX922	Bacterial cell, flagellum, basal structure
YX920	Bacterial cell, flagellum, NOS
YX921	Bacterial cell, flagellum, shaft
YX954	Bacterial cell, granular inclusion
YX901	Bacterial cell, macrocapsule
YX940	Bacterial cell, membrane, NOS
YX942	Bacterial cell, mesosome
YX902	Bacterial cell, microcapsule
YX952	Bacterial cell, nuclear material
YX930	Bacterial cell, pilum, NOS
YX941	Bacterial cell, protoplast membrane
YX953	Bacterial cell, ribosome
YX932	Bacterial cell, sex pilum
YX912	Bacterial cell wall, Gram —ve organism
YX911	Bacterial cell wall, Gram +ve organism
YX910	Bacterial cell wall, NOS
YX913	Bacterial cell wall, septum
YX914	Bacterial cell wall, surface convolutions
YX963	Bacterial spore, cortex
YX967	Bacterial spore, crystal
YX966	Bacterial spore, cytoplasm
YX965	Bacterial spore, cytoplasmic membrane
YX961	Bacterial spore, fore spore membrane
YX964	Bacterial spore, inner coat
YX962	Bacterial spore, outer coat
YX960	Bacterial spore structure, NOS
YX432	Band of microtubules, marginal
YX126	Barr body
YX455	Basal body, cilium or flagellum, not bacterial
YX203	Basal cell membrane, polarized cell
YX261	Basal infolding, cell membrane
YX859	Basal lamina, anchoring filaments
YX855	Basal lamina, discontinuous or incomplete
YX851	Basal lamina, epithelial cell or tissue

YX861	Basal lamina, inclusion consisting of cell process
YX862	Basal lamina, inclusion consisting of dense deposit
YX863	Basal lamina, inclusion in central location
YX864	Basal lamina, inclusion in subendothelial location
YX865	Basal lamina, inclusion in subepithelial location
YX860	Basal lamina, inclusion, NOS
YX856	Basal lamina, lamina densa component
YX858	Basal lamina, lamina rara externa component
YX857	Basal lamina, lamina rara interna component
YX852	Basal lamina, nonepithelial cell or tissue
YX850	Basal lamina, NOS
YX853	Basal lamina, specialized cell or tissue (T- . . .)
YX018	Basal region, polarized cell
YX922	Basal structure, bacterial flagellum
YX859	Basement membrane, anchoring filaments
YX855	Basement membrane, discontinuous
YX851	Basement membrane, epithelial cell or tissue
YX861	Basement membrane, inclusion consisting of cell process
YX862	Basement membrane, inclusion consisting of dense deposit
YX863	Basement membrane, inclusion in central location
YX864	Basement membrane, inclusion in subendothelial location
YX865	Basement membrane, inclusion in subepithelial location
YX860	Basement membrane, inclusion, NOS
YX856	Basement membrane, lamina densa component
YX858	Basement membrane, lamina rara externa component
YX857	Basement membrane, lamina rara interna component
YX852	Basement membrane, non-epithelial cell or tissue
YX850	Basement membrane, NOS
YX853	Basement membrane, specialized cell or tissue (T- . . .)
YX193	Beaded filamentous intranuclear body
YX356	Birbeck granule
YX111	Bleb, nuclear
YX527	Body, curvilamellar, within ER
YX193	Body, intranuclear, beaded filamentous type
YX194	Body, intranuclear, concentrically laminated
YX191	Body, intranuclear, filamentous
YX192	Body, intranuclear, granular with filamentous capsule
YX190	Body, intranuclear, NOS
YX195	Body, intranuclear, rod-shaped
YX643	Body, multivesicular, inclusion within
YX640	Body, multivesicular, NOS
YX626	Body, residual
YX195	Body, rod-shaped, intranuclear
YX640	Body, vesicle-containing

BRANCHING

YX713   Branching cristae, mitochondrion
YX708   "Bridge," mitochondrial

C

YX263   Canaliculus, intercellular
YX262   Canaliculus, intracellular
YX174   Cap, nucleolar
YX273   Caveola, NOS
YX274   Caveola, simple
YX210   Cell adhesion specialization, NOS
YX900   Cell capsule, prokaryotic, NOS
YX010   Cell, central region
YX280   Cell coat, NOS
YX563   Cell component (T-YX . . .), related to ER
YX950   Cell contents, prokaryotic, NOS
YX020   Cell, dividing, NOS
YX290   Cell envelope, distinctive form, NOS
YX033   Cell in mitosis, anaphase
YX032   Cell in mitosis, metaphase
YX030   Cell in mitosis, NOS
YX031   Cell in mitosis, prophase
YX034   Cell in mitosis, telophase
YX040   Cell in meiosis, NOS
YX201   Cell membrane, apical aspect, polarized cell
YX203   Cell membrane, basal aspect, polarized cell
YX202   Cell membrane, lateral aspect, polarized cell
YX200   Cell membrane, NOS
YX940   Cell membrane, prokaryotic, NOS
YX000   Cell, NOS
YX012   Cell, perinuclear region
YX013   Cell, peripheral region
YX014   Cell, polarized, apical region
YX018   Cell, polarized, basal region
YX017   Cell, polarized, infranuclear region
YX015   Cell, polarized, lateral region
YX016   Cell, polarized, supranuclear region
YX861   Cell process, inclusion within basal lamina
YX230   Cell process, NOS
YX740   Cell product or metabolite (F- . . .), intramitochondrial
YX181   Cell product (F- . . .), intranuclear
YX240   Cell surface process of distinctive morphology, NOS
YX561   Cell surface related to ER

YX806	Cell to cell relationship, characterized by absence of adhesion specializations
YX809	Cell to cell relationship, characterized by abundance of adhesion specializations
YX803	Cell to cell relationship, characterized by alternating areas of cell contact and separation
YX804	Cell to cell relationship, characterized by cell contact, separation minimal or absent
YX202	Cell to cell relationship, characterized by focal cell contact
YX805	Cell to cell relationship, characterized by interdigitation
YX808	Cell to cell relationship, characterized by presence of adhesion specializations
YX807	Cell to cell relationship, characterized by scantiness of adhesion specializations
YX801	Cell to cell repationship, characterized by cell separation, contact minimal or absent
YX800	Cell to cell relationship, distinctive, NOS
YX910	Cell wall, bacterial, NOS
YX914	Cell wall, bacterial, surface convolutions
YX291	Cell wall, eukaryotic
YX912	Cell wall, prokaryotic, Gram —ve organism
YX911	Cell wall, prokaryotic, Gram +ve organism
YX910	Cell wall, prokaryotic, NOS
YX913	Cell wall, prokaryotic, septum
YX219	Cement line of desmosome
YX221	Cementsome (T-01152)
YX863	Central inclusion within basal lamina
YX470	Central pair of microtubules, cilium or flagellum, not bacterial
YX010	Central region of cell
YX452	Central vesicle, centriole
YX173	Center, fibrillar, of nucleolus
YX452	Centriole, central vesicle
YX451	Centriole, microtubular subunit or triplet
YX450	Centriole, NOS
YX454	Centriole, satellite
YX457	Centriole, solitary microtubule
YX128	Centromere
YX011	Centrosome
YX277	Channel, micropinocytosis vermiformis
YX175	Channel system, nucleolar
YX384	Cholesterol crystal
YX752	Chondriosphere
YX127	Chromatid, NOS

CHROMATIN

YX123	Chromatin condensed
YX122	Chromatin extended
YX120	Chromatin, NOS
YX121	Chromatin, perinucleolar
YX160	Chromosome group, NOS
YX130	Chromosome, NOS
YX131	Chromosome pair 1
YX132	Chromosome pair 2
YX133	Chromosome pair 3
YX134	Chromosome pair 4
YX135	Chromosome pair 5
YX136	Chromosome pair 6
YX137	Chromosome pair 7
YX138	Chromosome pair 8
YX139	Chromosome pair 9
YX140	Chromosome pair 10
YX141	Chromosome pair 11
YX142	Chromosome pair 12
YX143	Chromosome pair 13
YX144	Chromosome pair 14
YX145	Chromosome pair 15
YX146	Chromosome pair 16
YX147	Chromosome pair 17
YX148	Chromosome pair 18
YX149	Chromosome pair 19
YX150	Chromosome pair 20
YX151	Chromosome pair 21
YX152	Chromosome pair 22
YX153	Chromosome pair 23
YX161	Chromosome pairs 1-3
YX162	Chromosome pairs 4-5
YX163	Chromosome pairs 6-12 and X
YX164	Chromosome pairs 13-15
YX165	Chromosome pairs 16-18
YX166	Chromosome pairs 19-20
YX167	Chromosome pairs 21-22 and Y
YX159	Chromosome, sex, NOS
YX15X	Chromosome X
YX15Y	Chromosome Y
YX161	Chromosomes, group A
YX162	Chromosomes, group B
YX163	Chromosomes, group C and X
YX164	Chromosomes, group D
YX165	Chromosomes, group E

YX166	Chromosomes, group F
YX167	Chromosomes, group G and Y
YX824	Chylomicron
YX465	Cilium, axial filament complex, NOS
YX470	Cilium, central pair of microtubules
YX469	Cilium, dynein arm of peripheral doublet
YX464	Cilium, membrane
YX460	Cilium, NOS
YX467	Cilium, peripheral doublet, subunit *a*
YX468	Cilium, peripheral doublet, subunit *b*
YX466	Cilium, peripheral microtubular doublet
YX456	Cilium, rootlet
YX461	Cilium, rudimentary
YX481	Cilium, sensory, olfactory (T-X8020)
YX463	Cilium, shaft
YX480	Cilium, specialized, NOS
YX490	Cilium, specialized subunit or derivative, NOS
YX116	Cisterna, perinuclear
YX523	Cisternae, confronting, of ER
YX552	Cisternal lumen, AER (SER)
YX572	Cisternal lumen, annulate lamella
YX522	Cisternal lumen, endoplasmic reticulum, NOS
YX532	Cisternal lumen, GER (RER)
YX212	Close junction
YX721	Close packing, cristae of mitochondrion
YX275	Coated vesicle
YX280	Coat of cell, NOS
YX721	Close packing, cristae of mitochondrion
YX842	Collagen fibrils, long spacing variety
YX841	Collagen fibrils, 64nm spacing
YX843	Collagen protofibrils
YX404	Combined actin-like and myosin-like filaments
YX931	Common pilum, bacterial
YX510	Complex, Golgi, NOS
YX812	Complex intercellular space
YX211	Complex, junctional, NOS
YX383	Complex lipid droplet
YX355	Complex melanin-containing granule
YX565	Concentric array, GER (RER)
YX724	Concentric orientation, cristae of mitochondrion
YX194	Concentrically laminated intranuclear body
YX123	Condensed chromatin
YX513	Condensing vacuole, Golgi complex
YX523	Confronting cisternae of ER

CONNECTIVE

YX840	Connective tissue fiber, NOS
YX830	Connective tissue matrix, NOS
YX847	Connective tissue microfibrils, NOS
YX208	Connexon
YX035	Constriction, anaphase
YX806	Contact relationship between cells, adhesion specializations absent or minimal
YX809	Contact relationship between cells, adhesion specializations abundant
YX808	Contact relationship between cells, adhesion specializations present
YX807	Contact relationship between cells, adhesion specializations scanty
YX803	Contact relationship between cells, alternating areas of cell contact and separation
YX801	Contact relationship between cells, contact minimal or absent
YX802	Contact relationship between cells, focal cell contact
YX805	Contact relationship between cells, interdigitation
YX804	Contact relationship between cells, separation absent or minimal
YX278	Content of endocytic membrane invagination (T-YX . . . or F- . . .)
YX279	Content of exocytic membrane invagination (F- . . .)
YX441	Continuous microtubules, mitotic spindle
YX401	Contractile apparatus, filaments, NOS
YX963	Cortex, bacterial spore
YX632	Crinophagocytic vacuole (F- . . .)
YX706	Cristae of mitochondrion
YX713	Cristae of mitochondrion, branching
YX721	Cristae of mitochondrion, closely packed
YX724	Cristae of mitochondrion, concentric orientation
YX720	Cristae of mitochondrion, distinctive pattern, NOS
YX710	Cristae of mitochondrion, distinctive shape, NOS
YX711	Cristae of mitochondrion, fenestrated
YX723	Cristae of mitochondrion, longitudinal orientation
YX715	Cristae of mitochondrion, prism-shaped
YX714	Cristae of mitochondrion, saccular
YX722	Cristae of mitochondrion, transverse orientation
YX712	Cristae of mitochondrion, tubular
YX725	Cristae of mitochondrion, zig-zag configuration
YX967	Crystal, bacterial spore
YX384	Crystal, cholesterol
YX834	Crystal, extracellular

YX733	Crystal, intramitochondrial
YX182	Crystal, intranuclear
YX311	Crystalline inclusion, cytoplasmic
YX182	Crystalline inclusion, intranuclear
YX384	Crystalline lipid
YX527	Curvilammellar body within ER
YX283	Cuticle of cell
YX631	Cytolysosome containing recognizable cytoplasmic organelle (T-YX . . .)
YX632	Cytolysosome containing secretion granule
YX630	Cytolysosome, NOS
YX966	Cytoplasm, bacterial spore
YX300	Cytoplasm, NOS
YX951	Cytoplasm, prokaryotic
YX405	Cytoplasmic filaments, distinctive arrangement, NOS
YX400	Cytoplasmic filaments, NOS
YX350	Cytoplasmic granule, NOS, distinctive, of specialized cell (T- . . .)
YX311	Cytoplasmic inclusion, crystalline
YX314	Cytoplasmic inclusion, filamentous
YX313	Cytoplasmic inclusion, granular
YX310	Cytoplasmic inclusion, NOS
YX312	Cytoplasmic inclusion, paracrystalline
YX300	Cytoplasmic matrix, NOS
YX965	Cytoplasmic membrane of bacterial spore
YX370	Cytoplasmic metabolite, structurally distinctive, NOS
YX430	Cytoplasmic microtubule, NOS
YX115	Cytoplasmic pseudo-inclusion within nucleus
YX590	Cytoplasmic synaptic specialization, NOS
YX320	Cytoplasmic vacuole, NOS, not related to GERL
YX630	Cytosegresome
YX433	Cytoskeleton
YX357	Cytosome, lamellated, as in surfactant-secreting cell

d

YX591	Dendritic spine apparatus
YX418	Dense body, cytoplasmic, with filament insertion
YX423	Dense bundles, intermediate filaments
YX346	Dense-cored synaptic vesicle
YX862	Dense deposit, inclusion within basal lamina

YX209	Dense zone, internal aspect of cell membrane, not desmosome
YX419	Dense zone, internal aspect of cell membrane, not desmosome, filament insertion
YX215	Desmosome
YX217	Desmosome, intracytoplasmic
YX221	Desmosome, mature, keratinocyte (T-01152)
YX219	Desmosome or hemidesmosome, extracellular dense component
YX226	Desmosome, septate
YX424	Desmosome-related tonofilaments
YX574	Diaphragm of fenestration, annulate lamella
YX253	Diaphragm of fenestration, endothelial (T-05130)
YX118	Diaphragm of nuclear pore
YX422	Diffuse tonofilaments
YX831	Diffusely mineralized extracellular matrix
YX435	Disc, adhesion type of parasite
YX222	Disc, intercalated, myocardium (T-33010)
YX020	Dividing cell, NOS
YX855	Discontinuous or incomplete basal or external lamina
YX405	Distinctive arrangement of cytoplasmic filaments, NOS
YX431	Distinctive arrangement of microtubules, NOS
YX560	Distinctive arrangement or relationship of endoplasmic reticulum, NOS
YX800	Distinctive cell to cell relationship, NOS
YX350	Distinctive cytoplasmic granule, specialized cell (T- . . .)
YX290	Distinctive form of cell envelope
YX281	Distinctive form of glycocalyx, NOS
YX580	Distinctive intracytoplasmic membrane system, not Golgi complex or ER
YX720	Distinctive pattern, mitochondrial cristae, NOS
YX710	Distinctive shape, mitochondrial cristae, NOS
YX240	Distinctive surface process, specialized cell, NOS
YX760	Dividing mitochondrion
YX734	DNA, intramitochondrial
YX466	Doublet, peripheral, cilium or flagellum, not bacterial
YX283	Droplet, lipid, complex
YX824	Droplet, lipid, extracellular
YX381	Droplet, lipid, homogeneous
YX382	Droplet, lipid, lamellated
YX380	Droplet, lipid, NOS
YX469	Dynein arm of peripheral doublet, cilium or flagellum, not bacterial

e

YX204	*E* face, fractured membrane
YX845	Elastic fiber, amorphous component
YX846	Elastic fiber, microfilamentous component
YX844	Elastic fiber, NOS
YX703	Electron transport particle
YX823	Endocrine secretion material, extracellular
YX341	Endocrine secretory granule, known content (F-...)
YX340	Endocrine secretory granule, NOS
YX342	Endocrine secretory granule undergoing exocytosis
YX343	Endocrine secretory granule undergoing exocytosis, known content (F-...)
YX278	Endocytic membrane invagination, content (T-YX... or F-...)
YX271	Endocytic membrane invagination, labile
YX567	Endoplasmic reticulum, agranular, aggregated
YX550	Endoplasmic reticulum, agranular or smooth
YX551	Endoplasmic reticulum, agranular or smooth, membrane
YX552	Endoplasmic reticulum, agranular or smooth, cisternal lumen
YX553	Endoplasmic reticulum, agranular or smooth, connection with other organelle (T-YX...)
YX568	Endoplasmic reticulum, agranular or smooth, striated muscle
YX526	Endoplasmic reticulum, amorphous intracisternal material
YX523	Endoplasmic reticulum, confronting cisternae
YX560	Endoplasmic reticulum, distinctive arrangement or relationship, NOS
YX530	Endoplasmic reticulum, granular
YX564	Endoplasmic reticulum, granular, aggregated, NOS
YX565	Endoplasmic reticulum, granular, concentric array
YX531	Endoplasmic reticulum, granular, membrane
YX566	Endoplasmic reticulum, granular, tubular array
YX533	Endoplasmic reticulum, granular or rough, connection with other organelle (T-YX...)
YX527	Endoplasmic reticulum, intracisternal curvilammelar body
YX525	Endoplasmic reticulum, intracisternal material
YX529	Endoplasmic reticulum, intracisternal material of known identity (F-...)
YX520	Endoplasmic reticulum, NOS
YX522	Endoplasmic reticulum, NOS, cisternal lumen
YX524	Endoplasmic reticulum, NOS, connection with other organelle (T-YX...)
YX528	Endoplasmic reticulum, NOS, intracisternal granule

YX521	Endoplasmic reticulum, NOS, membrane
YX527	Endoplasmic reticulum, periodic intracisternal material
YX561	Endoplasmic reticulum, related to cell surface
YX562	Endoplasmic reticulum, related to mitochondria
YX563	Endoplasmic reticulum, related to other cell component (T-YX . . .)
YX530	Endoplasmic reticulum, rough
YX550	Endoplasmic reticulum, smooth
YX360	Endothelial cell granule (T-05130)
YX253	Endothelial fenestration, diaphragm (T-05130)
YX250	Endothelial fenestration, NOS (T-05130)
YX251	Endothelial fenestration, with diaphragm (T-05130)
YX252	Endothelial fenestration, without diaphragm (T-05130)
YX254	Endothelial seive plate (T-05130)
YX111	Envelope, nuclear, evagination
YX114	Envelope, nuclear, inner membrane
YX115	Envelope, nuclear, invagination
YX110	Envelope, nuclear, NOS
YX112	Envelope, nuclear, outer membrane
YX113	Envelope, nuclear, outer membrane evagination
YX290	Envelope of cell, distinctive form, NOS
YX851	Epithelial cell or tissue, basal lamina
YX564	Ergastoplasm
YX520	ER, NOS
YX561	ER, related to cell surface
YX562	ER, related to mitochondrion
YX563	ER, related to other cell component (T-YX . . .)
YX122	Euchromatin
YX291	Eukaryotic cell wall
YX111	Evagination, nuclear envelope
YX113	Evagination, outer membrane of nuclear envelope
YX279	Exocytic membrane invagination, content (F- . . .)
YX272	Exocytic membrane invagination, labile
YX822	Exocrine secretion, extracellular phase
YX332	Exocrine secretory granule, known content (F- . . .)
YX333	Exocrine secretory granule, undergoing exocytosis
YX334	Exocrine secretory granule, undergoing exocytosis, known content (F- . . .)
YX331	Exocrine secretory granule, NOS
YX122	Extended chromatin
YX855	External lamina, discontinuous or incomplete
YX852	External lamina, nonepithelial cell or tissue
YX850	External lamina, NOS
YX853	External lamina, specialized cell or tissue (T- . . .)

YX835	Extracellular amorphous or granular material
YX834	Extracellular crystal
YX219	Extracellular dense component, desmosome or hemidesmosome
YX824	Extracellular lipid droplet
YX820	Extracellular material, NOS
YX831	Extracellular matrix material, diffusely mineralized
YX832	Extracellular matrix material, focally mineralized
YX833	Extracellular matrix material, nonmineralized
YX821	Extracellular metabolite or metabolic product (F-...)
YX823	Extracellular secretion material, following endocrine exocytosis
YX822	Extracellular secretion material, following exocrine exocytosis
YX810	Extracellular space, NOS

f

YX711	Fenestrated cristae, mitochondrion
YX573	Fenestration, annulate lamella
YX574	Fenestration, annulate lamella, diaphragm
YX253	Fenestration, endothelial, diaphragm (T-05130)
YX250	Fenestration, endothelial, NOS (T-05130)
YX251	Fenestration, endothelial, with diaphragm (T-05130)
YX252	Fenestration, endothelial, without diaphragm (T-05130)
YX374	Ferritin
YX741	Ferritin, intramitochondrial
YX840	Fiber, connective tissue, NOS
YX844	Fiber, elastic, NOS
YX845	Fiber, elastic, amorphous component
YX846	Fiber, elastic, microfilamentous component
YX173	Fibrillar center of nucleolus
YX836	Fibrin
YX119	Fibrous lamina, nucleus
YX491	Fibrous sheath, sperm tail (T-78180)
YX465	Filament complex, axial, of cilium
YX465	Filament complex, axial, of flagellum, not bacterial
YX418	Filament insertion into cytoplasmic dense body
YX419	Filament insertion into dense zone on internal aspect of cell membrane, not desmosome
YX424	Filament insertion into desmosome or hemidesmosome
YX417	Filament insertion, NOS
YX433	Filament-microtubule association
YX314	Filamentous cytoplasmic inclusion

FILAMENTOUS

YX191	Filamentous intranuclear body
YX183	Filamentous intranuclear inclusion
YX402	Filaments, 7nm, actin-like
YX421	Filaments, 9nm, intermediate
YX403	Filaments, 12nm, myosin-like
YX859	Filaments, anchoring, basal lamina
YX193	Filaments, beaded, intranuclear
YX404	Filaments, combined actin-like and myosin-like
YX401	Filaments, contractile apparatus, NOS
YX405	Filaments, cytoplasmic, distinctive arrangement, NOS
YX400	Filaments, cytoplasmic, NOS
YX421	Filaments, intermediate, 9nm, NOS
YX423	Filaments, intermediate, dense bundles
YX426	Filaments, intermediate, known composition (F-...)
YX183	Filaments, intranuclear
YX420	Filaments, structural, NOS
YX234	Filipodium
YX930	Fimbria, bacterial, NOS
YX920	Flagellum, bacterial, NOS
YX922	Flagellum, bacterial, basal structure
YX921	Flagellum, bacterial, shaft
YX465	Flagellum, not bacterial, axial filament complex, NOS
YX455	Flagellum, not bacterial, basal body
YX470	Flagellum, not bacterial, central pair of microtubules
YX469	Flagellum, not bacterial, dynein arm of peripheral microtubular doublet
YX464	Flagellum, not bacterial, membrane
YX462	Flagellum, not bacterial, NOS
YX466	Flagellum, not bacterial, peripheral microtubular doublet
YX467	Flagellum, not bacterial, peripheral microtubular doublet subunit *a*
YX468	Flagellum, not bacterial, peripheral microtubular doublet subunit *b*
YX456	Flagellum, not bacterial, rootlet
YX463	Flagellum, not bacterial, shaft
YX480	Flagellum, not bacterial, specialized, NOS
YX490	Flagellum, not bacterial, specialized subunit or derivative, NOS
YX630	Focal cytoplasmic degeneration, lysosome-related, NOS
YX832	Focally mineralized extracellular matrix
YX241	Fold, marginal, endothelial cell (T-01530)
YX242	Foot process, NOS, glomerular podocyte (T-71200)
YX243	Foot process, primary, glomerular podocyte (T-71200)
YX244	Foot process, secondary, glomerular podocyte (T-71200)

YX961	Fore spore membrane, bacterial
YX204	Fractured membrane, *E* face
YX206	Fractured membrane, intramembranous particle
YX207	Fractured membrane, particle array
YX205	Fractured membrane, *P* face
YX545	Free cytoplasmic polyribosome
YX541	Free cytoplasmic ribosome
YX582	Fusiform vesicle, as in transitional epithelium
YX275	Fuzzy vesicle

9

YX213	Gap junction
YX564	GER (RER) aggregate, NOS
YX565	GER (RER), concentric array
YX530	GER (RER), NOS
YX566	GER (RER), tubular array
YX500	GERL, NOS
YX242	Glomerular podocyte, foot process, NOS (T-71200)
YX243	Glomerular podocyte, primary foot process (T-7120)
YX244	Glomerular podocyte, secondary foot process (T-71200)
YX245	Glomerular podocyte, slit pore (T-71200)
YX281	Glycocalyx, distinctive form
YX280	Glycocalyx, NOS
YX372	Glycogen, α pattern
YX373	Glycogen, β pattern
YX186	Glycogen, intranuclear
YX371	Glycogen, NOS
YX510	Golgi complex, apparatus or system, NOS
YX516	Golgi complex, inclusion within
YX511	Golgi membrane
YX512	Golgi saccule
YX513	Golgi vacuole
YX514	Golgi vesicle, NOS
YX313	Granular cytoplasmic inclusion
YX564	Granular endoplasmic reticulum, aggregated, NOS
YX532	Granular endoplasmic reticulum, cisternal lumen
YX565	Granular endoplasmic reticulum, concentric array
YX533	Granular endoplasmic reticulum, connection with other organelle (T-YX . . .)
YX531	Granular endoplasmic reticulum membrane
YX530	Granular endoplasmic reticulum, NOS
YX566	Granular endoplasmic reticulum, tubular array

GRANULAR

YX835	Granular extracellular material
YX954	Granular inclusion, prokaryotic
YX192	Granular intranuclear body with filamentous capsule
YX835	Granular or amorphous extracellular material
YX651	Granule, acrosomal (T-78170)
YX356	Granule, Birbeck type
YX355	Granule, complex, melanin-containing
YX350	Granule, cytoplasmic, distinctive, NOS, specialized cell (T-...)
YX360	Granule, endothelial cell (T-05130)
YX125	Granule, interchromatin
YX528	Granule, intracisternal of ER, NOS
YX732	Granule, intramitochondrial
YX361	Granule, keratohyaline
YX357	Granule, lamellated, as in surfactant-secreting cell
YX356	Granule, Langerhans type
YX626	Granule, lipofuscin
YX355	Granule, melanin-containing, complex
YX354	Granule, melanogenic, completely melanized
YX353	Granule, melanogenic, incompletely melanized
YX352	Granule, melanogenic, nonmelanized
YX351	Granule, melanogenic, NOS
YX364	Granule, membrane-coating, amorphous
YX363	Granule, membrane-coating, laminated
YX362	Granule, membrane-coating, NOS
YX335	Granule, mucus
YX344	Granule, neurosecretory type
YX564	Granule, Nissl
YX124	Granule, perichromatin
YX652	Granule, proacrosomal (T-78170)
YX341	Granule, secretory, endocrine, known content (F-...)
YX343	Granule, secretory, endocrine, known content (F-...) undergoing exocytosis
YX340	Granule, secretory, endocrine, NOS
YX342	Granule, secretory, endocrine, undergoing exocytosis
YX332	Granule, secretory, exocrine, known content (F-...)
YX334	Granule, secretory, exocrine, known content (F-...) undergoing exocytosis
YX331	Granule, secretory, exocrine, NOS
YX333	Granule, secretory, exocrine, undergoing exocytosis
YX188	Granule, secretory, intranuclear
YX330	Granule, secretory, NOS
YX336	Granule, zymogenic
YX360	Granule, Weibel-Palade type (T-01530)

h

YX413	*H* zone, sarcomere (T-13000)
YX246	Hair, sensory (T-YX840, T-YX890)
YX218	Hemidesmosome
YX425	Hemidesmosome, attachment plaque
YX219	Hemidesmosome, extracellular dense component
YX424	Hemidesmosome, filament insertion
YX123	Heterochromatin
YX621	Heterolysosome
YX300	Hyaloplasm, NOS

i

YX412	*I* band, sarcomere (T-13000)
YX311	Inclusion, cytoplasmic crystalline
YX314	Inclusion, cytoplasmic, filamentous
YX313	Inclusion, cytoplasmic, granular
YX310	Inclusion, cytoplasmic, NOS
YX312	Inclusion, cytoplasmic, paracrystalline
YX862	Inclusion, dense deposit type, within basal lamina
YX182	Inclusion, intranuclear, crystalline
YX183	Inclusion, intranuclear, filamentous
YX184	Inclusion, intranuclear, lamellar
YX180	Inclusion, intranuclear, NOS
YX185	Inclusion, intranuclear, tubular
YX954	Inclusion, prokaryotic, granular
YX863	Inclusion with basal lamina, central location
YX861	Inclusion within basal lamina, consisting of cell process
YX862	Inclusion within basal lamina, dense deposit type
YX864	Inclusion within basal lamina, subendothelial location
YX865	Inclusion within basal lamina, subepithelial location
YX516	Inclusion within Golgi complex
YX866	Inclusion within mesangial matrix (T-71290)
YX731	Inclusion within mitochondrial matrix, NOS
YX730	Inclusion within mitochondrion, NOS
YX 643	Inclusion within multivesicular body
YX855	Incomplete basal or external lamina
YX261	Infolding, cell membrane, basal
YX017	Infranuclear region, polarized cell
YX964	Inner coat, bacterial spore
YX702	Inner membrane, mitochondrion

YX114	Inner membrane, nuclear envelope
YX705	Inner space, mitochondrion
YX418	Insertion of filaments into cytoplasmic dense body
YX419	Insertion of filaments into dense zone on internal aspect of cell membrane, not desmosome
YX424	Insertion of filaments into desmosome or hemidesmosome
YX417	Insertion of filaments, NOS
YX222	Intercalated disc, myocardium (T-33101)
YX263	Intercellular canaliculus
YX812	Intercellular space, complex or labyrinthine
YX811	Intercellular space, NOS
YX125	Interchromatin granule
YX805	Interdigitating cell to cell relationship
YX642	Internal vesicles, multivesicular body
YX423	Intermediate filament bundles, dense
YX421	Intermediate filaments, 9nm, NOS
YX426	Intermediate filaments, known composition (F-...)
YX214	Intermediate junction
YX101	Interphase nucleus
YX442	Interzonal microtubules, mitotic spindle
YX262	Intracellular canaliculus
YX527	Intracisternal curvilamellar body of ER
YX528	Intracisternal granule of ER, NOS
YX526	Intracisternal material, amorphous, within ER
YX529	Intracisternal material, known identity, within ER (F-...)
YX525	Intracisternal material, NOS, within ER
YX527	Intracisternal material, periodic, within ER
YX217	Intracytoplasmic desmosome
YX265	Intracytoplasmic lumen
YX580	Intracytoplasmic membrane system, distinctive, not Golgi complex or ER
YX740	Intramitochondrial cell metabolite (F-...)
YX733	Intramitochondrial crystal
YX734	Intramitochondrial DNA
YX741	Intramitochondrial ferritin
YX732	Intramitochondrial granule
YX730	Intramitochondrial inclusion, NOS
YX742	Intramitochondrial lipid
YX735	Intramitochondrial ribosome
YX193	Intranuclear body, beaded
YX194	Intranuclear body, concentrically laminated
YX191	Intranuclear body, filamentous
YX192	Intranuclear body, granular with filamentous capsule
YX190	Intranuclear body, NOS

YX195	Intranuclear body, rod shaped
YX181	Intranuclear cell product (F- . . .)
YX182	Intranuclear crystal or crystalline inclusion
YX115	Intranuclear cytoplasmic pseudo-inclusion
YX183	Intranuclear filament or filamentous inclusion
YX186	Intranuclear glycogen
YX182	Intranuclear inclusion, crystalline
YX183	Intranuclear inclusion, filamentous
YX184	Intranuclear inclusion, lamellar
YX180	Intranuclear inclusion, NOS
YX185	Intranuclear inclusion, tubular
YX187	Intranuclear lipid
YX184	Intranuclear membrane lamellae
YX189	Intranuclear mitochondrion
YX188	Intranuclear secretory granule
YX185	Intranuclear tubule or tubular inclusion
YX271	Invagination, endocytic
YX278	Invagination, endocytic, known content (T-YX . . . or F- . . .)
YX272	Invagination, exocytic
YX279	Invagination, exocytic, known content (F- . . .)
YX260	Invagination, fixed or stable, cell membrane
YX270	Invagination, labile, cell membrane
YX115	Invagination, nuclear envelope
YX002	Isolated subcellular structure, following fractionation procedure

j

YX212	Junction, close type
YX215	Junction, desmosome type
YX213	Junction, gap type
YX214	Junction, intermediate type
YX226	Junction, septate
YX212	Junction, tight type
YX211	Junctional complex, NOS

k

YX120	Karyoplasm
YX110	Karyotheca
YX427	Keratin, mature
YX361	Keratohyaline granule

KINETOCHORE

YX129	Kinetochore
YX770	Kinetoplast, NOS
YX455	Kinetosome
YX460	Kinocilium, NOS

L

YX271	Labile membrane invagination, endocytic
YX272	Labile membrane invagination, exocytic
YX270	Labile membrane invagination, NOS
YX812	Labyrinthine intercellular space
YX572	Lamella, annulate, cisternal lumen
YX574	Lamella, annulate, diaphragm of fenestration
YX573	Lamella, annulate, fenestration
YX571	Lamella, annulate, membrane
YX570	Lamella, annulate, NOS
YX184	Lamellar intranuclear inclusion
YX357	Lamellated granule, as in surfactant-secreting cell
YX382	Lamellated lipid droplet
YX235	Lamellipodium
YX859	Lamina, basal, anchoring filaments
YX855	Lamina, basal, discontinuous or incomplete
YX860	Lamina, basal, inclusion within, NOS
YX850	Lamina, basal, NOS
YX851	Lamina, basal, epithelial cell or tissue
YX852	Lamina, basal, nonepithelial cell or tissue
YX853	Lamina, basal or external, specialized cell or tissue (T- . . .)
YX856	Lamina densa component, basal lamina
YX850	Lamina, external, NOS
YX855	Lamina, external or basal, discontinuous or incomplete
YX852	Lamina, external or basal, nonepithelial cell or tissue
YX853	Lamina, external or basal, specialized cell or tissue (T- . . .)
YX119	Lamina, fibrous, of nucleus
YX858	Lamina rara externa component, basal lamina
YX857	Lamina rara interna component, basal lamina
YX363	Laminated membrane-coating granule
YX356	Langerhans granule
YX202	Lateral cell membrane, polarized cell
YX015	Lateral region, polarized cell
YX807	Limited cell contact with adhesion specialization
YX804	Limited cell contact without adhesion specialization
YX384	Lipid, crystalline
YX383	Lipid droplet, complex

YX824	Lipid droplet, extracellular
YX381	Lipid droplet, homogeneous
YX382	Lipid droplet, lamellated
YX380	Lipid droplet, NOS
YX742	Lipid, intramitochondrial
YX187	Lipid, intranuclear
YX626	Lipofuscin granule
YX723	Longitudinal orientation, cristae of mitochondrion
YX842	Long spacing collagen
YX552	Lumen, cisternal, AER (SER)
YX572	Lumen, cisternal, annulate lamella
YX522	Lumen, cisternal, endoplasmic reticulum, NOS
YX532	Lumen, cisternal, GER (RER)
YX265	Lumen, intracytoplasmic
YX822	Luminal secretion material
YX627	Lysosome, adhesion specialization
YX623	Lysosome-derived myelin figure
YX650	Lysosome, male germ cell (T-78180)
YX602	Lysosome matrix
YX601	Lysosome membrane
YX600	Lysosome, NOS
YX610	Lysosome, primary, NOS
YX620	Lysosome, secondary, NOS
YX625	Lysosome, secondary, undergoing exocytosis
YX622	Lysosome, secondary, with distinctive content (T-YX . . . or F-. . .)
YX624	Lysosome, secondary, with ferritin content
YX623	Lysosome, secondary, with laminated content

m

YX414	*M* line, sarcomere
YX901	Macrocapsule, bacterial cell
YX215	Macula adherens
YX650	Male germ cell, lysosome (T-78180)
YX432	Marginal band of microtubules
YX241	Marginal fold, endothelial cell (T-05130)
YX830	Matrix, connective tissue, NOS
YX300	Matrix, cytoplasmic, NOS
YX831	Matrix, extracellular, diffusely mineralized
YX832	Matrix, extracellular, focally mineralized
YX833	Matrix, extracellular, nonmineralized
YX732	Matrix granule, mitochondrial

MATRIX

YX731	Matrix inclusion, mitochondrial, NOS
YX602	Matrix, lysosomal
YX854	Matrix, mesangial (T-71290)
YX866	Matrix, mesangial, inclusion within (T-71290)
YX662	Matrix, microbody or peroxisome
YX705	Matrix, mitochondrial
YX040	Meiotic cell, NOS
YX355	Melanin-containing granule, complex
YX354	Melanin granule
YX351	Melanogenic granule, NOS
YX354	Melanosome, completely melanized
YX353	Melanosome, incompletely melanized
YX352	Melanosome, nonmelanized
YX551	Membrane, AER (SER)
YX571	Membrane, annulate lamella
YX961	Membrane, bacterial fore spore
YX941	Membrane, bacterial protoplast
YX200	Membrane, cell, NOS
YX940	Membrane, cell, prokaryotic, NOS
YX464	Membrane, cilium or flagellum, not bacterial
YX364	Membrane-coating granule, amorphous
YX363	Membrane-coating granule, laminated
YX362	Membrane-coating granule, NOS
YX965	Membrane, cytoplasmic, bacterial spore
YX521	Membrane, endoplasmic reticulum, NOS
YX206	Membrane, fractured, intramembranous particle
YX207	Membrane, fractured, particle array
YX531	Membrane, GER (RER)
YX511	Membrane, Golgi complex
YX261	Membrane infolding, base of cell
YX702	Membrane, inner mitochondrial
YX703	Membrane, inner mitochondrial, particle
YX114	Membrane, inner, nuclear envelope
YX260	Membrane invagination, fixed or stable, NOS
YX271	Membrane invagination, labile, endocytic
YX272	Membrane invagination, labile, exocytic
YX270	Membrane invagination, labile, NOS
YX184	Membrane lamellae, intranuclear
YX581	Membrane lamellae, photoreceptor
YX601	Membrane, lysosome
YX661	Membrane, microbody or peroxisome
YX701	Membrane, outer mitochondrial
YX112	Membrane, outer, nuclear envelope
YX113	Membrane, outer, nuclear envelope, evagination

YX200	Membrane, plasma, NOS
YX201	Membrane, polarized cell, apical aspect
YX203	Membrane, polarized cell, basal aspect
YX202	Membrane, polarized cell, lateral aspect
YX284	Membrane receptor (F- . . .)
YX210	Membrane specialization, cell adhesion type
YX225	Membrane specialization, postsynaptic
YX224	Membrane specialization, presynaptic
YX223	Membrane specialization, NOS, synaptic
YX641	Membrane surrounding multivesicular body
YX580	Membrane system, intracytoplasmic, not Golgi complex or ER
YX854	Mesangial matrix (T-71290)
YX866	Mesangial matrix inclusion (T-71290)
YX942	Mesosome, bacterial
YX370	Metabolite, cytoplasmic, structurally distinctive, NOS
YX740	Metabolite, intramitochondrial, NOS
YX743	Metabolite, known constitution (F- . . .), intramitochondrial
YX821	Metabolite or metabolic product, extracellular (F- . . .)
YX032	Metaphase, mitotic cell
YX104	Metaphase nucleus
YX105	Metaphase plate
YX666	Microbody adhesion specialization
YX662	Microbody matrix
YX661	Microbody membrane
YX660	Microbody, NOS
YX664	Microbody nucleoid, amorphous
YX663	Microbody nucleoid, NOS
YX665	Microbody nucleoid, periodic
YX902	Microcapsule, bacterial cell
YX847	Microfibrils, connective tissue, NOS
YX846	Microfilamentous component, elastic fiber
YX277	Micropinocytosis vermiformis channel
YX273	Micropinocytotic vesicle, NOS
YX466	Microtubular doublets, peripheral, cilium or flagellum, not bacterial
YX451	Microtubular subunit or triplet, centriole
YX471	Microtubule, solitary, axonemal complex
YX457	Microtubule, solitary, centriole
YX434	Microtubules associated with cell organelle (T-YX . . .)
YX433	Microtubules associated with cytoplasmic filaments
YX470	Microtubules, central pair, cilium or flagellum, not bacterial
YX441	Microtubules, continuous, mitotic spindle
YX430	Microtubules, cytoplasmic, NOS
YX431	Microtubules, distinctive arrangement, NOS

MICROTUBULES

YX442	Microtubules, interzonal, mitotic spindle
YX432	Microtubules, marginal band
YX232	Microvillous border
YX231	Microvillus
YX036	Midbody, telophase
YX707	Mitochondrial adhesion specialization
YX750	Mitochondrial aggregation within cytoplasm, NOS
YX751	Mitochondrial association with other cell component (T-YX . . .)
YX708	Mitochondrial "bridge"
YX706	Mitochondrial cristae
YX713	Mitochondrial cristae, branching
YX721	Mitochondrial cristae, closely packed
YX724	Mitochondrial cristae, concentric orientation
YX720	Mitochondrial cristae, distinctive pattern, NOS
YX710	Mitochondrial cristae, distinctive shape, NOS
YX711	Mitochondrial cristae, fenestrated
YX723	Mitochondrial cristae, longitudinal orientation
YX715	Mitochondrial cristae, prism-shaped
YX714	Mitochondrial cristae, saccular
YX722	Mitochondrial cristae, tranversely orientated
YX712	Mitochondrial cristae, tubular
YX725	Mitochondrial cristae, zig-zag configuration
YX733	Mitochondrial crystal
YX734	Mitochondrial DNA
YX741	Mitochondrial ferritin
YX732	Mitochondrial granule
YX730	Mitochondrial inclusion, NOS
YX742	Mitochondrial lipid
YX705	Mitochondrial matrix
YX731	Mitochondrial matrix inclusion, NOS
YX702	Mitochondrial membrane, inner
YX701	Mitochondrial membrane, outer
YX703	Mitochondrial membrane particle
YX740	Mitochondrial metabolite
YX562	Mitochondrial relationship to ER
YX735	Mitochondrial ribosome
YX705	Mitochondrial space, inner
YX704	Mitochondrial space, outer
YX760	Mitochondrion in division
YX189	Mitochondrion, intranuclear
YX700	Mitochondrion, NOS
YX033	Mitotic cell, anaphase
YX032	Mitotic cell, metaphase

YX030	Mitotic cell, NOS
YX031	Mitotic cell prophase
YX034	Mitotic cell, telophase
YX102	Mitotic nucleus, NOS
YX440	Mitotic spindle, NOS
YX443	Mitotic spindle, pole
YX335	Mucus granule
YX643	Multivesicular body, inclusion
YX642	Multivesicular body, internal vesicles
YX640	Multivesicular body, NOS
YX641	Multivesicular body, surrounding membrane
YX623	Myelin figure, lysosome-derived or myelinosome
YX401	Myofilaments
YX403	Myosin-like filaments, 12nm

n

YX344	Neurosecretory granule
YX213	Nexus
YX564	Nissl granule or substance
YX833	Nonmineralized extracellular matrix
YX111	Nuclear bleb
YX190	Nuclear body, NOS
YX191	Nuclear body, simple
YX111	Nuclear envelope, evagination
YX114	Nuclear envelope, inner membrane
YX115	Nuclear envelope, invagination
YX110	Nuclear envelope, NOS
YX112	Nuclear envelope, outer membrane
YX113	Nuclear envelope, outer membrane evagination
YX119	Nuclear fibrous lamina
YX952	Nuclear material, prokaryotic
YX117	Nuclear pore apparatus
YX118	Nuclear pore diaphragm
YX120	Nuclear sap
YX664	Nucleoid, amorphous, microbody or peroxisome
YX663	Nucleoid, NOS, microbody or peroxisome
YX665	Nucleoid, periodic, microbody or peroxisome
YX174	Nucleolar cap
YX175	Nucleolar channel system
YX173	Nucleolinus
YX171	Nucleolonema
YX173	Nucleolus, fibrillar center

NUCLEOLUS

YX170	Nucleolus, NOS
YX172	Nucleolus, pars amorpha or fibrosa
YX171	Nucleolus, pars granulosa
YX106	Nucleus, anaphase
YX115	Nucleus, cytoplasmic pseudo-inclusion
YX101	Nucleus, interphase
YX104	Nucleus, metaphase
YX102	Nucleus, mitotic, NOS
YX100	Nucleus, NOS
YX103	Nucleus, prophase
YX107	Nucleus, telophase

O

YX212	Occluding junction
YX362	Odland body
YX481	Olfactory sensory cilium (T-X8020)
YX962	Outer coat, bacterial spore
YX710	Outer membrane, mitochondrion
YX112	Outer membrane, nuclear envelope
YX113	Outer membrane, nuclear envelope, evagination
YX482	Outer segment, retinal photoreceptor (T-XX610)
YX704	Outer space, mitochondrial

P

YX205	P face, fractured membrane
YX312	Paracrystalline cytoplasmic inclusion
YX435	Parasite adhesion disc
YX292	Parasite pellicle
YX172	Pars amorpha or fibrosa, nucleolus
YX171	Pars granulosa, nucleolus
YX207	Particle array, fractured membrane
YX703	Particle, electron transport
YX206	Particle, intramembranous, fractured membrane
YX703	Particle, mitochondrial inner membrane
YX244	Pedicel, glomerular podocyte (T-71200)
YX292	Pellicle, as in protozoal parasite
YX124	Perichromatin granule
YX116	Perinuclear cisterna
YX012	Perinuclear region of cell
YX116	Perinuclear space

YX121	Perinucleolar chromatin
YX527	Periodic material within ER cisterna
YX665	Periodic nucleoid, microbody or peroxisome
YX466	Peripheral microtubular doublet, cilium or flagellum, not bacterial
YX469	Peripheral microtubular doublet, cilium or flagellum, not bacterial, dynein arm
YX467	Peripheral microtubular doublet, cilium or flagellum, not bacterial, subunit *a*
YX468	Peripheral microtubular doublet, cilium or flagellum, not bacterial, subunit *b*
YX013	Peripheral region of cell
YX666	Peroxisomal adhesion specialization
YX662	Peroxisome matrix
YX661	Peroxisome membrane
YX660	Peroxisome, NOS
YX663	Peroxisome nucleoid
YX664	Peroxisome nucleoid, amorphous
YX665	Peroxisome nucleoid, period
YX621	Phagolysosome or phagosome
YX271	Phagosome
YX581	Photoreceptor membrane lamellae, NOS
YX482	Photoreceptor, retinal, outer segment (T-XX610)
YX931	Pilum, bacterial, common pilum
YX930	Pilum, bacterial, NOS
YX932	Pilum, bacterial, sex pilum
YX425	Plaque, attachment, desmosome or hemidesmosome
YX200	Plasmalemma or plasma membrane, NOS
YX780	Plastid, NOS
YX105	Plate, metaphase
YX242	Podocyte, glomerular, foot process, NOS (T-71200)
YX243	Podocyte, glomerular, primary foot process (T-71200)
YX244	Podocyte, glomerular, secondary foot process or pedicel (T-71200)
YX245	Podocyte, glomerular, slit pore (T-71200)
YX201	Polarized cell, apical cell membrane
YX014	Polarized cell, apical region
YX203	Polarized cell, basal cell membrane
YX018	Polarized cell, basal region
YX017	Polarized cell, infranuclear region
YX202	Polarized cell, lateral cell membrane
YX015	Polarized cell, lateral region
YX016	Polarized cell, supranuclear region
YX443	Pole, mitotic spindle

YX546	Polyribosome, attached to GER membrane
YX547	Polyribosome, attached to outer nuclear membrane
YX545	Polyribosome, free in cytoplasm
YX544	Polyribosome, NOS
YX117	Pore apparatus, nuclear
YX118	Pore, nuclear, diaphragm
YX245	Pore, slit type, glomerular podocyte (T-71200)
YX225	Post-synaptic membrane specialization
YX352	Premelanosome
YX224	Pre-synaptic membrane specialization
YX243	Primary foot process, glomerular podocyte (T-71200)
YX610	Primary lysosome, NOS
YX715	Prism-shaped cristae, mitochondrion
YX652	Proacrosomal granule (T-78170)
YX453	Procentriole
YX230	Process of cell, NOS
YX240	Process, specialized cell, distinctive surface morphology, NOS
YX922	Prokaryotic cell, basal structure, flagellum
YX900	Prokaryotic cell, capsule, NOS
YX931	Prokaryotic cell, common pilum
YX950	Prokaryotic cell, contents, NOS
YX951	Prokaryotic cell, cytoplasm
YX920	Prokaryotic cell, flagellum, NOS
YX961	Prokaryotic cell, fore spore membrane
YX954	Prokaryotic cell, granular inclusion
YX901	Prokaryotic cell, macrocapsule
YX940	Prokaryotic cell, membrane, NOS
YX942	Prokaryotic cell, mesosome
YX902	Prokaryotic cell, microcapsule
YX952	Prokaryotic cell, nuclear material
YX930	Prokaryotic cell, pilum, NOS
YX941	Prokaryotic cell, protoplast membrane
YX953	Prokaryotic cell, ribosome
YX932	Prokaryotic cell, sex pilum
YX921	Prokaryotic cell, shaft of flagellum
YX912	Prokaryotic cell wall, Gram —ve organism
YX911	Prokaryotic cell wall, Gram +ve organism
YX910	Prokaryotic cell wall, NOS
YX913	Prokaryotic cell wall, septum
YX963	Prokaryotic spore, cortex
YX967	Prokaryotic spore, crystal
YX966	Prokaryotic spore, cytoplasm
YX965	Prokaryotic spore, cytoplasmic membrane
YX961	Prokaryotic spore, fore spore membrane

YX964	Prokaryotic spore, inner coat
YX962	Prokaryotic spore, outer coat
YX960	Prokaryotic spore structure, NOS
YX031	Prophase, mitotic cell
YX103	Prophase nucleus
YX843	Protofibrils, collagen
YX941	Protoplast membrane, bacterial or prokaryotic
YX115	Pseudo-inclusion, cytoplasmic, within nucleus

r

YX284	Receptor, membrane (F- . . .)
YX014	Region, apical, polarized cell
YX018	Region, basal, polarized cell
YX010	Region, central, of cell
YX017	Region, infranuclear, polarized cell
YX015	Region, lateral, polarized cell
YX012	Region, perinuclear, of cell
YX013	Region, peripheral, of cell
YX106	Region, supranuclear, polarized cell
YX806	Relationship between cells, characterized by absence of adhesion specializations
YX809	Relationship between cells, characterized by abundance of adhesion specializations
YX803	Relationship between cells, characterized by alternating areas of cell contact and separation
YX804	Relationship between cells, characterized by cell contact, separation minimal or absent
YX801	Relationship between cells characterized by cell separation, contact minimal or absent
YX802	Relationship between cells, characterized by focal cell contact
YX805	Relationship between cells, characterized by interdigitation
YX808	Relationship between cells, characterized by presence of adhesion specializations
YX807	Relationship between cells, characterized by scantiness of adhesion specializations
YX800	Relationship between cells, distinctive, NOS
YX564	RER (GER), aggregated, NOS
YX565	RER (GER), concentric array
YX530	RER (GER), NOS
YX566	RER (GER), tubular array
YX626	Residual body

RETICULUM

YX550	Reticulum, endoplasmic, agranular
YX567	Reticulum, endoplasmic, agranular, aggregated, NOS
YX552	Reticulum, endoplasmic, agranular, cisternal lumen
YX553	Reticulum, endoplasmic, agranular, connection with other organelle (T-YX . . .)
YX551	Reticulum, endoplasmic, agranular, membrane
YX568	Reticulum, endoplasmic, agranular, striated muscle
YX526	Reticulum, endoplasmic, amorphous intracisternal material
YX523	Reticulum, endoplasmic, confronting cisternae
YX560	Reticulum, endoplasmic, distinctive arrangement or relationship, NOS
YX530	Reticulum, endoplasmic, granular
YX564	Reticulum, endoplasmic, granular, aggregated, NOS
YX532	Reticulum, endoplasmic, granular, cisternal lumen
YX565	Reticulum, endoplasmic, granular, concentric array
YX533	Reticulum, endoplasmic, granular, connection with other organelle (T-YX . . .)
YX531	Reticulum, endoplasmic, granular, membrane
YX566	Reticulum, endoplasmic, granular, tubular array
YX527	Reticulum, endoplasmic, intracisternal curvilamellar body
YX529	Reticulum, endoplasmic, intracisternal material, known identity (F- . . .)
YX525	Reticulum, endoplasmic, intracisternal material, NOS
YX520	Reticulum, endoplasmic, NOS
YX522	Reticulum, endoplasmic, NOS, cisternal lumen
YX524	Reticulum, endoplasmic, NOS, connection with other organelle (T-YX . . .)
YX528	Reticulum, endoplasmic, NOS, intracisternal granule
YX521	Reticulum, endoplasmic, NOS, membrane
YX527	Reticulum, endoplasmic, periodic intracisternal material
YX561	Reticulum, endoplasmic, related to cell surface
YX562	Reticulum, endoplasmic, related to mitochondrion
YX563	Reticulum, endoplasmic, related to other cell component (T-YX . . .)
YX568	Reticulum, sarcoplasmic
YX482	Retinal photoreceptor, outer segment (T-XX610)
YX276	Rhopheocytotic vesicle
YX542	Ribosome, attached to GER (RER) membrane
YX543	Ribosome, attached to outer nuclear membrane
YX541	Ribosome, free in cytoplasm
YX735	Ribosome, intramitochondrial
YX540	Ribosome, NOS
YX953	Ribosome, prokaryotic
YX195	Rod-shaped intranuclear body

YX456	Rootlet of cilium or flagellum, not bacterial
YX530	Rough endoplasmic reticulum
YX565	Rough endoplasmic reticulum, aggregated, NOS
YX532	Rough endoplasmic reticulum, cisternal lumen
YX566	Rough endoplasmic reticulum, concentric array
YX533	Rough endoplasmic reticulum, connection with other organelle (T-YX . . .)
YX567	Rough endoplasmic reticulum, tubular array
YX461	Rudimentary cilium
YX235	Ruffle of cell surface

S

YX714	Saccular cristae, mitochondrion
YX512	Saccule, Golgi complex
YX120	Sap, nuclear
YX411	Sarcomere, *A* band
YX413	Sarcomere, *H* zone
YX412	Sarcomere, *I* band
YX414	Sarcomere, *M* line
YX410	Sarcomere pattern, NOS
YX415	Sarcomere, *Z* line
YX568	Sarcoplasmic reticulum
YX454	Satellite of centriole
YX244	Secondary foot process, glomerular podocyte (T-71200)
YX620	Secondary lysosome, NOS
YX622	Secondary lysosome with distinctive content (T-YX . . . or F- . . .)
YX624	Secondary lysosome with ferritin content
YX623	Secondary lysosome with laminated content
YX625	Secondary lysosome, undergoing exocytosis
YX341	Secretory granule, endocrine, known content (F- . . .)
YX343	Secretory granule, endocrine, known content (F- . . .), undergoing exocytosis
YX340	Secretory granule, endocrine, NOS
YX342	Secretory granule, endocrine, undergoing exocytosis
YX332	Secretory granule, exocrine, known content (F- . . .)
YX334	Secretory granule, exocrine, known content (F- . . .), undergoing exocytosis
YX331	Secretory granule, exocrine, NOS
YX333	Secretory granule, exocrine, undergoing exocytosis
YX188	Secretory granule, intranuclear
YX330	Secretory granule, NOS

SEIVE

YX254	Seive plate, endothelial (T-05130)
YX481	Sensory cilium, olfactory (T-X8020)
YX246	Sensory hair (T-YX840, T-YX890)
YX226	Septate junction or desmosome
YX913	Septum, prokaryotic cell wall
YX567	SER (AER), aggregated, NOS
YX553	SER (AER), connection with other organelle (T-YX . . .)
YX550	SER (AER), NOS
YX126	Sex chromatin
YX159	Sex chromosome, NOS
YX15X	Sex chromosome X
YX15Y	Sex chromosome Y
YX932	Sex pilum, bacterial
YX921	Shaft, bacterial flagellum
YX463	Shaft, cilium or flagellum, not bacterial
YX491	Sheath, fibrous, sperm tail (T-78180)
YX624	Siderosome
YX274	Simple caveola
YX191	Simple nuclear body
YX471	Singlet or solitary axonemal microtubule
YX245	Slit pore, glomerular podocyte (T-71200)
YX567	Smooth endoplasmic reticulum, aggregated, NOS
YX552	Smooth endoplasmic reticulum, cisternal lumen
YX553	Smooth endoplasmic reticulum, connection with other organelle (T-YX . . .)
YX551	Smooth endoplasmic reticulum, membrane
YX550	Smooth endoplasmic reticulum, NOS
YX471	Solitary microtubule, axonemal complex
YX457	Solitary microtubule, centriole
YX705	Space, mitochondrial, inner
YX704	Space, mitochondrial, outer
YX116	Space, perinuclear
YX480	Specialized cilium or flagellum, not bacterial, NOS
YX490	Specialized subunit or derivative, cilium or flagellum, not bacterial, NOS
YX491	Sperm tail, fibrous sheath (T-78180)
YX440	Spindle, mitotic, NOS
YX443	Spindle, mitotic, pole
YX963	Spore cortex, bacterial
YX967	Spore crystal, bacterial
YX966	Spore cytoplasm, bacterial
YX965	Spore cytoplasmic membrane, bacterial
YX964	Spore inner coat, bacterial
YX962	Spore outer coat, bacterial

YX960	Spore structure, bacterial, NOS
YX233	Stereocilium
YX232	Striated border
YX420	Structural filaments, NOS
YX002	Subcellular structure, isolated by fractionation technique
YX001	Subcellular structure, NOS
YX864	Subendothelial inclusion, basal lamina
YX865	Subepithelial inclusion, basal lamina
YX467	Subunit *a,* peripheral doublet, cilium or flagellum, not bacterial
YX468	Subunit *b,* peripheral doublet, cilium or flagellum, not bacterial
YX451	Subunit, microtubular triplet, centriole
YX016	Supranuclear region, polarized cell
YX914	Surface convolutions, bacterial cell wall
YX357	Surfactant-secreting cell, lamellated granule
YX223	Synaptic membrane specialization, NOS
YX225	Synaptic membrane specialization, post-synaptic
YX224	Synaptic membrane specialization, pre-synaptic
YX590	Synaptic specialization, cytoplasmic, NOS
YX346	Synaptic vesicle, dense cored
YX345	Synaptic vesicle, NOS

t

YX264	T tubule, striated muscle
YX626	Telolysosome
YX036	Telophase, midbody
YX034	Telophase, mitotic cell
YX107	Telophase nucleus
YX212	Tight junction
YX423	Tonofibrils, NOS
YX422	Tonofilaments, diffuse
YX421	Tonofilaments, NOS
YX424	Tonofilaments, related to desmosome or hemidesmosome
YX515	Transport or transitional vesicle, Golgi complex
YX722	Transverse orientation, cristae of mitochondrion
YX569	Triad, striated muscle
YX567	Tubular array, GER (RER)
YX712	Tubular cristae, mitochondrion
YX185	Tubule, intranuclear
YX264	Tubule, T type, striated muscle

UNCLASSIFIED 79

U

YXX00 Unclassified ultrastructural features
YX236 Uropod

V

YX513 Vacuole, condensing, Golgi complex
YX632 Vacuole, crinophagocytic (F- . . .)
YX320 Vacuole, cytoplasmic, NOS, not related to GERL
YX237 Vermipodium
YX653 Vesicle, acrosomal (T-78180)
YX452 Vesicle, central, centriole
YX275 Vesicle, coated
YX640 Vesicle-containing or multivesicular body
YX582 Vesicle, fusiform, as in transitional epithelium
YX275 Vesicle, fuzzy
YX514 Vesicle, Golgi, NOS
YX515 Vesicle, Golgi, transport or transitional type
YX642 Vesicle, internal, multivesicular body
YX273 Vesicle, micropinocytotic, NOS
YX276 Vesicle, rhopheocytotic
YX346 Vesicle, synaptic, dense-cored
YX345 Vesicle, synaptic, NOS

W

YX291 Wall of cell, eukaryotic
YX360 Weibel-Palade granule (T-05130)

X

YX15X X Chromosome

Y

YX15Y Y Chromosome

Z

YX416   Z line material
YX415   Z line, sarcomere
YX725   Zig-zag configuration, cristae of mitochondrion
YX214   Zonula adherens
YX212   Zonula occludens
YX336   Zymogen granule

appendix

proposed revised listing of m-6 codes

600   **Karyotype abnormalities**

60000	Karyotype abnormality, NOS
60010	XXY Karyotype
60011	XO Karyotype
60012	XYY Karyotype
60040	Alteration of chromosome number, NOS
	Aneuploidy, NOS
60041	Hyperdiploidy
60042	Trisomy
60043	Endoreduplication
60044	Polyploidy
60045	Hypodiploidy
60046	Monosomy
	Deletion, whole chromosome

601   **Structural chromosome alterations**

60100	Alteration of chromosome structure, NOS
60110	Deletion of short arm
60120	Philadelphia chromosome, Ph1 present
60130	Philadelphia chromosome, Ph1 absent
60140	Deletion of long arm
60150	Lengthening of short arm
60160	Lengthening of long arm
60170	Isochromosome for short arm
60180	Isochromosome for long arm
60190	Chromosome break
60200	Chromatid break
60210	Chromosome inversion, NOS

60220	Pericentric inversion
60230	Paracentric inversion
60240	Ring chromosome
60250	Chromosome fragment

603 Centromere alterations

60300	Acentric chromosome
60301	Dicentric chromosome
60302	Tricentric chromosome

604 Translocations

60400	Translocation, NOS
60410	Translocation, centric fusion
60420	Translocation, reciprocal
60430	Translocation, Robertsonian

605 Abnormal chromosome bandings

60500	Abnormal chromosome banding, NOS

620 Distinctive cytologic morphologies

62000	Distinctive cytologic morphology, NOS
62010	Anuclear cell
62011	Anuclear squame
62030	Foam cell
62040	Glycogenic cell
62100	Fusiform cell
62110	Tadpole cell
62120	Folded cell
62130	Tear drop cell
62140	Signet ring cell
62150	Smudge cell
62160	Pancake cell
62170	Navicular cell
62200	Megaconial abnormality
62210	Target fibers
62220	Contraction bands

PROPOSED REVISED LISTING OF M-6 CODES

62230	Rosenthal fiber
62240	Sarcoplasmic masses
62300	Satellitosis
62310	Neuronophagia
62320	Gemistocyte
	Gemistocytic astrocyte
62330	Alzheimer change
	Alzheimer type II glial cell
62400	Hematoxylin body
62410	Russell body
62500	Megalocyte
	Macrocyte
	Giant cell
62510	Multinucleate giant cell
	Warthin-Finkeldey giant cell
62520	Microcyte
62530	Alteration, syncytial
	Syncytial formation
62600	Vacuolation
	Vacuolization
62700	Positive-stain reaction, NOS
62701	Eosinophilic
62702	Basophilic
62703	Amphophilic
62704	Metachromatic
62710	Sudanophilic
62720	Osmiophilic
62730	Schiff positive

640 Atypia etc.

64000	Atypia cytologic, NOS
	N.B. 5th digit
	Various topographic variants
64010	Atypia, squamous cell
64020	Atypia, columnar cell
64030	Atypia, transitional cell
64040	Atypia, inflammatory
	Alteration of cellular material, inflammatory
64050	Atypia, suspicious for malignancy
64060	Atypia, koilocytotic
64100	Pleomorphism
	Polymorphism

64200	Dyskaryosis
64210	Macronucleus
	Karyomegaly
64211	Karyopyknosis
	Pyknosis
64212	Micronucleus
64213	Anisokaryosis
64214	Chromatolysis
64220	Nuclear/cytoplasmic ratio, abnormal, NOS
64221	Nuclear/cytoplasmic ratio increased
64222	Nuclear/cytoplasmic ratio decreased
64300	Abnormal numbers of nuclei
	Multinucleate cell, NOS
64301	Binucleate cell
64310	Perinuclear halo
64320	Hyperchromatism
	Hyperchromasia
64321	Hypochromatism
	Hypochromasia
64322	Achromasia
64330	Hypersegmentation
	Hypersegmented nucleus
64331	Hyposegmentation
	Hyposegmented nucleus

650   Cellular hormonal patterns

65000	Cellular hormonal pattern, normal
65010	Cellular hormonal pattern, abnormal
65020	Estrogen effect, NOS
65030	No estrogen effect present
	Estatrophy
65040	Low level estrogen effect present
65050	Moderate level estrogen effect present
65060	High level estrogen effect present
65070	Progesterone effect present
65080	Pregnancy pattern
65090	Telatrophy
	Parabasal cells predominate